Ayurvedic Healing

Ayurvedic Healing

FRENA GRAY-DAVIDSON

Keats Publishing

Chicago   New York   San Francisco   Lisbon   London   Madrid   Mexico City
Milan   New Delhi   San Juan   Seoul   Singapore   Sydney   Toronto

Library of Congress Cataloging-in-Publication Data

Davidson, Frena Gray.
  Ayurvedic healing / by Frena Gray-Davidson.
    p. cm.
  Includes bibliographical references and index.
  ISBN 0-658-01147-2
    1. Medicine, Ayurvedic.   I. Title.

R605 .D385 2001
615.5'3—dc21   2001035784

Keats Publishing

*A Division of The **McGraw-Hill** Companies*

1 2 3 4 5 6 7 8 9 0   DOC/DOC   0 9 8 7 6 5 4 3 2 1

ISBN: 0-658-01147-2

This book was designed and set in Bembo by Laurie Young
Printed and bound by R. R. Donnelley—Crawfordsville

Cover design by Laurie Young
Cover illustration by Margaret Chodos-Irvine

McGraw-Hill books are available at special quantity discounts to use as premiums and sales promotions, or for use in corporate training programs. For more information, please write to the Director of Special Sales, Professional Publishing, McGraw-Hill, Two Penn Plaza, New York, NY 10121-2298. Or contact your local bookstore.

The purpose of this book is to educate. It is sold with the understanding that the publisher and author shall have neither liability nor responsibility for any injury caused or alleged to be caused directly or indirectly by the information contained in this book. While every effort has been made to ensure their accuracy, the book's contents should not be construed as medical advice. Each person's health needs are unique. To obtain recommendations appropriate to your particular situation, please consult a qualified health care provider.

This book is printed on acid-free paper.

This book is dedicated to that great army of light and hope, those who look after the young, the old, the sick, and the dying— and who know that love is the key, the purpose, and the solution.

May you all have a really, *really* good night's sleep tonight!

CONTENTS

ACKNOWLEDGMENTS

I am very grateful to Dr. Deepak Chopra who has single-handedly done so much to bring Ayurveda to westerners in an understandable, helpful, cross-cultural way. Without his teaching, writing this book would have been impossible. He has shown me a way to cut through the jargon and the metaphors and bring clarity to a complex subject, and I deeply appreciate that.

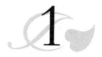

The Science of Life

*"I ignorant, unknowing, seek knowledge
From those seers who may know."*

—RIG VEDA

A yurveda, like traditional Chinese medicine, has a very long history. Ayurveda has its roots in one of the greatest civilizations of the ancient world, that of the Indus River Valley.

It is thought that this civilization developed as a result of a great migration of people from the northwestern regions of Asia to the Indus Valley. These people, known as the Aryans, brought a sophisticated religious, spiritual, and healing tradition with them. Great cities arose in the fertile Indus Valley, with sophisticated and well-developed systems of living that would be acceptable to people living now. The Indus Valley people had working sewage systems consisting of great pipes running beneath paved streets. Their houses had hot water systems and under-the-floor heating. They traveled and they met great scholars and philosophers from all the trading kingdoms of Asia. Ideas, science, and religion flourished in the Indus Valley.

It was out of this coming together that a sophisticated science came to be. The science of life: Ayurveda.

Although we might think of Ayurveda as solely a system of health and medicine, its real meaning is much more broad. In fact, it extends to every aspect of life and consciousness. It is a system of knowledge about the human being at all levels. It deals with the whole person, from the material body of flesh, blood, and bone to the heart and the soul.

The name *Ayurveda* comes from two separate words in Sanskrit, the ancient language of the Aryan peoples of India. *Ayur* derives from a word meaning "life," while *veda* means "science or knowledge." Unlike Western allopathic medicine, Ayurveda is not merely a study of symptoms of disease—it is a holistic system that includes the study of wellness and harmony. It is an ancient exploration of the ways in which we live as complete beings at all levels of existence—physical, mental, emotional, energetic, and spiritual.

Ayurveda was not built on studying the dead nor on the listing of symptoms of sickness, but on learning how well people manifest good health. Its study was wholeness. This school of knowledge contains a thorough understanding of herbal medicine—Ayurveda was treating asthma and respiration problems with the plant ephedra over two thousand years ago, well before Western medicine came up with the use of ephedrine for the same problems. It also includes systems—yoga and meditation—for creating harmony within, recognizing that it is in the lack of such harmony that most illnesses have their roots. In medical knowledge, Ayurveda included surgery, the study of poisons, obstetrics, and gynecology.

2

Ayurveda is also a profound system of preventive medicine. It recognizes that human beings fit into a number of well-established groups that indicate certain inclinations toward disease when their lives are disrupted and lack harmony. As part of preventive medicine, it encompasses diet, exercise, and the particular foods most suitable for each type of person. It does not assume, as Western allopathic medicine does, that human beings are basically the same.

Ayurveda recognizes the important differences between types of people and the profound ways in which each can be helped—or harmed—by the food they eat and the way it is cooked. Like traditional Chinese medicine, Ayurveda believes that human beings are part of the natural world and that we find our perfect way of being from staying conscious of this truth.

Ayurveda's ancient writings teach that nature and its workings, its seasons, its weather, and its manifestations in the world around us will deeply affect the ways in which we all live. Therefore, Ayurvedic physicians teach that it is also important to focus on how humans may best live in harmony with the natural world.

As we begin to look at the ways in which Ayurveda describes people and their conditions, you will notice that many of its terms are drawn from the terminology of the natural world. This is because the natural world was all that was known when Ayurveda had its origins. Human beings had not turned themselves into people who lived separated from and largely ignorant of the natural world. They merely dwelt in nature and only knew themselves to be part of it.

You will find words of climate, weather, and environment

3

used to describe the processes of wellness and illness. They are terms that are both metaphors and accurate descriptions of processes. Just as traditional Chinese medicine draws much of its terminology from the natural world, Ayurveda also sees us in this world, interacting with nature and our environment. We are an essential part of it, living in relationship with it. When we forget this, or live with little or no awareness of the natural world, our disharmony is born.

Many great philosophical teachings agree that we are one with the universe. Some Ayurvedic tools for achieving a state of harmony include herbal medicines, aromatic and essential oils, sandalwood, frankincense, rose, and spices such as cinnamon and cardamom used for medicinal purposes. Other forms of Ayurvedic treatment are derived from the use of precious and semiprecious stones for their healing abilities, while other treatments may extend to special massages using milk, sweet oils, and honey.

Although Ayurveda is considered a holistic system for complete wellness, it does offer a wide range of specific treatments for specific conditions that can afflict many of us, even though we may try to attain perfect wellness. Ayurveda also includes teachings that encourage spiritual attainment. This book will outline all these systems as well as provide a practical introduction to the ways in which you may use Ayurvedic knowledge for your own health and well-being. Since Ayurveda has become much more recognized throughout the United States, it will not be hard to get any of the Ayurvedic supplies listed in the resources section of this book.

The most well-known practitioner of Ayurveda is Dr. Deepak Chopra, M.D., who is both a western allopathic doctor and an Ayurvedic practitioner. He has probably done the most public work to bring this ancient healing tradition to general notice. Now, there are several Ayurvedic schools and foundations in the United States, including that of Dr. Vesant Lad in Albuquerque, New Mexico. A more complete listing of such contacts can be found in the resources section.

The history of Ayurveda says that the *Rishis*—sages and visionaries—received cosmic knowledge of Ayurveda from the gods or a "cosmic consciousness" while meditating in the sacred areas of the Himalayas. The word *Rishi* comes from the Sanskrit word meaning "seer." In Hindu tradition, the Rishis are regarded as the ancestors from whom sprang the great priestly families of Hinduism. Tradition states that they draw their knowledge directly from the heavens as a result of their meditations. The Rishis then passed on their knowledge by oral teachings, from spiritual teacher to disciple, and these teachings did not become written down until the creation of the Vedas, the first works to be created in the sacred language of Sanskrit. The most important of these writings are considered to be the *Rig Veda* and the *Arthava Veda*. The *Rig Veda*, which is commonly dated to about 1300 B.C. by present-day scholars, is the first commentary on ritual, devotion, and well-being to appear on the Indian subcontinent. It is expressed in a series of songs, prayers, and instructions for ritual that are not easy for even Sanskrit scholars to fully comprehend. For the average reader, much of the *Rig Veda* is incomprehensible and it certainly does not form a tightly organized system of medical and healing understanding.

There is every reason to believe that both traditional Chinese medicine and Ayurvedic systems began their development at about the same time and that they have the same roots.

5

Both share certain approaches to holistic health, such as utilizing forms of acupuncture, massage, and energy medicine. Both refer to the nature of a disease and its particular symptoms by utilizing the same concepts of cooling and heating. Both categorize foods as neutral, heating, and cooling. Both also depend upon medicinal herbs, often the same herbs. Both use the Five Element System as a basic way of classifying diseases. Because of these commonalties, it is easy to conclude that Ayurveda and traditional Chinese medicine may have come from a common source.

This keen observation comes from my own period of fifteen years of study in both Indian and Chinese cultures. It is not acknowledged by either culture nor written of in any publicly available documents. It is, however, part of both Chinese and Indian sacred oral teachings. This conclusion, which is at odds with traditional Ayurvedic teaching, is presented here because it has validity.

The first medical document from ancient Egyptian medical texts, known to scholars as the *Ebers Papyrus,* is dated about 1500 B.C. In other words, the great healing systems of Asia were developing on a time line similar to that on the African continent, and the three civilizations were linked by trade routes that provided the necessary interconnectedness. This unacknowledged interconnection of three great civilizations can be deduced from the ways in which they developed their healing systems with certain common threads. When several major systems with similarities develop at about the same time, we have to assume that they are interlinked in some way. It was this rich network of connection across the trade routes that allowed the sharing of knowledge.

The *Rig Veda* is much less an actual health and treatment text than the first traditional Chinese medicine text, *The Yellow Emperor's Classic of Internal Medicine*. This is an original classic of traditional Chinese medicine and is traditionally claimed by the Chinese to be five thousand years old; however, modern scholars have dated it to about 1000 B.C. *The Yellow Emperor's Classic* is a sophisticated and detailed medical text, still used today as a basis for understanding health in human beings. Readers unfamiliar with the concepts of traditional Chinese medicine will get a clear idea of its basic concepts from reading this text. The fact that it dates to about five hundred years later than the *Rig Veda* allows for an additional five hundred years of processing the systems of medical knowledge.

Secret Taoist teachings, shared with me by a Taoist master in Hong Kong when I spent five years there studying traditional Chinese medicine and acupuncture, say that Beings of Light who came from the skies brought knowledge of traditional Chinese medicine. Sanskrit tradition, however, states that the gods themselves gave knowledge of Ayurveda to the Hindus. These somewhat similar accounts suggest a common mythic or historic origin for the teachings.

Another common thread is that each of the two medical systems contains knowledge that, properly applied, enables the human being to become an enlightened being. Ayurveda certainly contains this as a basic part of its yoga and meditative teachings. It clearly states that its essence is to bring about the uniting of human with divine consciousness. Ayurveda teaches that without this relationship, human beings cannot be fully healthy. Secret Taoist teachings proclaim the same possibilities in acupuncture. The Taoist mystics say that the meridian system of the human body has certain mystical points that can be activated by energy alone, without the use of acupuncture needles. Manipulating these secret points can enable the human being to become fully enlightened.

In about 800 B.C., the first Ayurvedic medical school was founded in India by Punavarsu Atreya, regarded as a great sage who received his knowledge directly from the gods themselves, especially from the god Indra, the god of healing. Hindu mythology says that the god Indra received his knowledge from divine physicians who had been taught by Brahma the Creator of the Universe. Atreya was said to have gone on a great quest to find such teachings and, after he had succeeded, he taught the principles of Ayurveda all over India to share and propagate the divine knowledge of healing. The sage Atreya created special symposia to spread these teachings, and he had six especially brilliant followers, one of whom—Agnivesa—wrote down Atreya's teachings in the work known as the *Agnivesa Tantra*.

This and other treatises on Ayurveda were later collected and further developed by Charaka, a scholar who lived sometime between 700 and 800 B.C. His work was summarized in the treatise known as the *Charaka Samhita*, which contains references to 1,500 plants, about 350 of which he identified as medically valuable. His treatise is still regarded as one of the great classics of Ayurveda and is still used as a tool for treatment today.

This gathering of medical knowledge was said to derive from a meeting of great sages and medical men from all over the Indus Valley. This meeting was set to discuss the problems of illness and disease and to find solutions for them, so that human beings could live to achieve their fullest spiritual potential.

During the same time period, surgery was being developed as a necessary adjunct to Ayurvedic herbal treatment, to be used when all else failed. Developing separately, surgery of various kinds was nevertheless included in the whole body of work known as Ayurveda. Surgery had several specialties included in its discipline, from gynecology and obstetric to what we might call plastic surgery. The great sage of surgery was the scholar and surgeon Susruta, and it was he who wrote the major Ayurvedic treatise on surgery known as *Susruta Samhita.* This text is still regarded as one of the great treatises of Ayurveda and is still used today by Ayurvedic practitioners.

Surgery would have been an ordeal in those ancient times if the people of the Indus Valley had not used the anesthetic substance soma. To this day, no one can say what soma actually was. Theories include that it was something derived from either the opium poppy, magic mushrooms, or even *Cannabis sativa,* which grows wild in this part of India. Whatever soma was, its legendary existence indicates that surgeons might well have had substances available to make operations painless.

After its founding, the influences of Ayurveda spread far and wide along the trading routes. It certainly strongly influenced Tibetan and maybe traditional Chinese medicine to the Far East and farther west to Arabia. Medicine was highly developed in Arabia, and it was the great teachings of the Arab physicians—notably the eleventh-century philosopher and scientist Avicenna—that began to bring light into the medical darkness of still-primitive Europe.

Ayurveda entered its own dark ages after British merchants effectively seized power in India and gradually annexed most of it for the British government, adding India's riches and wealth of materials to the vast commercial warehouse known as the British Empire. As well as making Indians second-class citizens in their own country, the British closed down all Ayurvedic schools in 1833. They dismissed Ayurvedic medicine as superstitious nonsense.

Fortunately, Ayurveda survived the formal closure of schools and was restored to its honored position as India's own natural healing choice once the British had been kicked out of India and Indian freedom restored. Now, there are schools training Ayurvedic physicians all over India and throughout the world, including the United States, and it has become an ancient healing system whose approach and basic belief system is very much in tune with that of the medical consumers of the twenty-first century. Ayurveda has proven that it is here to stay.

2

The Whole Human Being

When we read or hear about the Ayurvedic ideas, it has a surprisingly modern sound to its essential teachings. This is why many people insist on referring to this three-thousand-year-old system as "new age." What they really mean is that we have developed our thinking about health and wellness in ways that have moved beyond symptom and treatment. We have arrived at the point at which we are finally ready to understand healing systems that acknowledge that we become "dis-eased" and healed at the level of our highest and deepest being—the atomic or energy level.

In spite of the seemingly cumbersome jargon of Sanskrit terms, there is little that is totally strange to us in Ayurveda. The basic concepts that make the most sense to us are those that refer to harmony. We are all familiar with the concept that ideal health is not merely a state of being well, but it is something more proactive—the state of maximum harmony. We all seek and need harmony, and by creating harmony for ourselves we also create wellness. The traditional texts of Ayurveda indicate that our ultimate state of well-being comes about when we also nurture a capacity to identify and develop the divine in ourselves. Ayurveda is a health system that recognizes our ultimate possible being and directs us in ways that we can achieve it. Ayurveda takes us beyond the merely emotional and material toward the sacred center of life. This sacred center is not seen as separate, but is intrinsic. These are familiar ideas to us; ideas which are also found in homeopathy and in traditional Chinese medicine. Where Ayurveda differs is in its extension to states of soul and consciousness.

Our ultimate wellness, says Ayurveda, comes from fully achieving our ultimate potential as human beings. That inevitably involves our divine nature as well as our body, our emotions, our temperament, and the ways in which all our parts evolve. Ayurveda also recognizes that our intrinsic nature is to be in harmony. Living in total harmony is seen as our well-being and natural destiny. This has also become a very familiar idea to us in the early part of the twenty-first century. Most people no longer have any difficulty accepting that health is not just a matter of symptoms and disease. It is a matter of our entire life at all its levels, including how we think and feel about things. We know that feelings can give rise to disease. Most of us instinctively know that health is deeply involved with feelings and attitudes. Ask a sick person why they are sick, and they often have a deep sense of what gave rise to their illness. Something happened that allowed the roots of illness to take hold.

People often feel the truth of their illnesses. Disharmony —in mind, body, or spirit—eventually gives rise to actual disease. In other words, a change or disruption to the natural flow of energy in the human being is the forerunner to the appearance of physical ailments. Thus women who develop breast cancer can inevitably point to a serious shock or disruption they experienced about eighteen months before the manifestation of their cancer. Only Western medicine itself seems to be continuously surprised by this concept as study after study confirms it for allopathic physicians. One recent study affirmed that hostile people have a higher incidence of heart disease and heart attacks. Hippocrates identified in his writings about health the importance that emotions had on the ability to stay healthy and to heal.

Even diseases that do not seem like energy events—Alzheimer's, for example—follow an extended series of life stresses and are often manifested after a major shock, accident, or event of loss. This reminds us that even diseases we think of as mysterious or unsolved have their origins in the energy system and the ways in which life is lived. Taken at its purest and most powerful level, this knowledge takes us far.

It tells us that not only is it our basic nature to be whole but also that we may "re-achieve" wholeness. No matter what our disease, no matter what doctors say about it, we may achieve wholeness again. This is what Deepak Chopra refers to as "quantum healing," a healing possible because our entire nature is energy.

Oddly enough, it is the insurance industry that has observed this concept best. The actuary risk table assigns a number value to various life events—marriage, divorce, change of address, new job, getting fired, and so on—and predicts serious accident or illness for the individual who scores high in any of these areas. Yet, you will never find these life events referred to in the medical chart of a person who has had a heart attack or an outbreak of cancer. It is as if a great and profound truth has been pushed aside.

Ayurveda recognizes our ultimate possibilities and has many ways to help us come to them. The disciplines of Ayurveda —its treatments and its fundamental spiritual teachings of yoga and meditation—are what help us move from our states of imperfection toward our natural state of perfection. We, along with the conditions of the universe, create our states of "disease," and Ayurveda teaches us how to remove the toxins of mind and body so that we may come to harmony. This is especially true today when the basic nature of our universe has become so corrupted and polluted.

What brings us into harmony and wholeness is balance. Our whole organism is constantly seeking balance and constantly trying to come back into balance. It is our natural center. Deepak Chopra talks of how our body has many thermostats and how we constantly seek to return to balance in each and to have harmony in this immensely complex system of ours. The imbalances that may develop in us—through our bad habits, our environment, or life events—are called *vikriti*. These vikriti have the power to push us toward accumulated imbalance. Someone who doesn't get enough sleep because of personal habits—staying out late, taking stimulants—will begin to change throughout their whole system. Emotional life changes—physical, spiritual—deteriorate under the influence of vikriti. When we live out of harmony,

14

it is inevitable and unavoidable that we shall pay for this in our physical, mental, and emotional health bodies. We have energy accounts and when we overdraw them, our systems manifest illness.

Ayurveda has studied closely over the ages exactly how illnesses develop. There are six stages to the process:

1. Accumulation—energy from one of the three *doshas* (this term will be defined later) begins to gather through a growing imbalance, which begins purely at an energy level. Something happens that is registered only in the energy system of the body, but it is from this shock or loss or change that effects ripple outward.

2. Aggravation—the excess of one dosha energy causes it to violate its normal controls.

3. Dissemination—the excess energy invades the whole body.

4. Localization—the dosha gathers in a part of the body where it should not be. Typically, it gathers at a site already vulnerable. These vulnerable sites come about for the following reasons: heredity, karma, unresolved emotions, physical and psychological trauma, previous illnesses, and addictions.

5. Manifestation—physical symptoms begin to arise in that place.

6. Disruption—full-blown disease appears.

The first three stages are apparent only to the person who is reasonably observant of his or her own body. The signs are subtle, and not usually available for a real diagnosis. There might be

15

vague aches and pains or some internal discomfort too diffuse to really identify. These might even become quite demanding—internal spasms, strong feelings of pain—but still yielding few discernible clues to the instruments of Western medicine. Often, this is the stage at which a person intuitively knows there is something wrong, but there is no clear evidence.

Disruptions of harmony may be felt, but often they cannot be measured by external instruments. Too frequently they may be dismissed as psychosomatic by a Western physician, but an Ayurvedic doctor would recognize what was happening and begin intervention. Balance can be restored relatively easily in the first three stages of illness development through the use of diet, exercise, and attention to the routines of daily living. This is why it is so valuable for people to know their basic Ayurvedic type and the kinds of life patterns that support their type.

CHAKRA SYSTEM

The chakras are major energy centers found in a line along the center of the body beginning at the root chakra at the sexual organs and extending up to the top of the head, known as the "crown chakra." Although the terminology is different, these closely correspond with the meridian system in traditional Chinese medicine, which says that each major organ of the body has its own energy system that may be depleted or enhanced by life and by medicinal intervention. The energy centers of each chakra are often referred to more as spiritual energy than as functioning organ energy, but we may regard them as both.

In the West, we reveal a familiarity with such concepts when we refer to our heart as if it were an emotional center, as much as we may think of it as an actual physical organ of the body. In fact, if we receive an emotional blow, we can even feel the pain or heaviness of that emotional blow as a physical actuality in our body. Someone who has lost a love will often feel an actual pain or ache in the heart area. It is because of this that we are not far from understanding the dual concept expressed in the chakra system. We know about "gut feelings." We even say, "I know it in my bones." So, we understand that there is a wisdom within the material body that is not merely related to matters of the flesh or physical symptoms.

17

Root Chakra

This is the first chakra, and it usually is considered to be midway between the sexual organ and anus; it is associated with the uterus and the prostate gland. It is from this chakra that the kundalini energy spiral begins. This is the energy that is regarded as a sign of great spiritual awakening.

There are many traditional yoga and tantric practices that are aimed at raising kundalini energy so that it rises up through all the chakras and through the crown chakra. We can think of this as a great spiritual clearing of the whole energy system.

Splenic Chakra

The second chakra is called splenic chakra by some teachers. This is associated with the testes and ovaries. It is this level at which wounding is experienced in sexual abuse. The energy of this chakra can be restored by herbs like coriander and fennel that are warming and counteract deep spiritual shock and physical trauma.

Solar Plexus

The third chakra is called the solar plexus. This is the level at which we receive a great deal of psychic, intuitive, or gut-feeling information about the world and the people in it that we meet. This vulnerable area can be protected by folding the hands across the center of the belly, a useful tactic when dealing with hostile people. The solar plexus is associated with the liver and the adrenal glands and can be effectively helped by the herbs goldenseal and lemon balm.

Heart Chakra

The fourth chakra is known as the heart chakra, the center of emotional feeling. When we are out of touch with our feelings, we can reconnect with them by folding our hands over our heart and sitting quietly. This chakra is connected with the thymus gland and the heart, the thymus being the regulator of the immune system.

We can stimulate the thymus gland by tapping or patting our chest. This is sometimes seen as an automatic response to shock. This movement will enhance your heart energy and help you to deal with the situation. Rose essential oil is the great opener of the heart chakra, and it brings healing to a wounded heart.

Throat Chakra

The fifth chakra is the throat chakra. This has been long over-looked by people who assume that it is somehow the least important of the chakras. However, it is the major linkage between the heart and the head. Tibetans regard it is as one of the three minds that operate in human attitudes. This is because of its association with speaking out and expressing opinions, attitudes, and feelings.

It is the most likely chakra to be wounded in sexual abuse, because of the impossibility often imposed on abused children to "not speak out." Because of this, it is through opening the throat chakra—as in singing, for example—that healing can be found. Associated with the thyroid gland, this chakra is "tonified" by the use of cloves and vervain.

Third Eye

The sixth chakra is known as the "Third Eye." This is found midway between the eyes at brow level and is associated with the pituitary gland.

It is this gland that is thought to be directly influenced by spiritual enlightenment. Sandalwood oil and the herb elecampane are supporters of the sixth chakra.

Crown Chakra

The seventh chakra or the crown chakra is regarded as the height of the spiritual energy system within the human body. This chakra must be open for full spiritual realization to take place. It takes a level of spiritual maturity for the crown chakra to open. At death, the soul of an enlightened person exits only through the crown chakra, and it is believed that this is the way we connect with the higher energies of the universe.

This chakra is associated with the pineal gland and aided by herbs like gotu kola and nutmeg essential oil. The chakra system does not end there, however. Most spiritual teachers in the Hindu tradition teach that there are as many as twelve chakras, five of which extend beyond the body into the human energy system.

In Middle English, the word *whole* shares a common root with the word *health* and also the word *healed*. In our modern world, it is useful for us to remind ourselves how closely these concepts used to be linked. There is a deep connection between the idea of wellness and wholeness. This connection is really the spiritual.

To this day, there are many societies in the world where sickness is recognized as a manifestation of spiritual uneasiness— "dis-ease"—and must be approached both through the body and the spirit.

This is the basic stance of Ayurveda. It acknowledges any level at which "dis-ease-iness" may occur. Diseases do not work in a vacuum. They occur in human beings. Even in perfect balance, each human being is different. Therefore, wholeness is to be found when we know who this individual person is and could be when well. One of the clearest signs of a whole human being is when everything is in its harmonic flow. Energies flow through the balanced chakras, encouraging flow of blood, air, chemicals, and gases through the body to all organs. Energies flow through the emotional range—anger, grief, and joy. Nothing is blocked. Nothing is in excess. This flow of physical and emotional energies makes up a whole person.

Ayurvedic exercises encourage proper flow between the physical and emotional energies. Yoga is a series of complex body movements designed to increase flexibility—or muscle flow—and it allows no space for blockage and stifling in the body. With blockage comes disease and disharmony. *Prana*, or breathing exercises, are all about taking in the right amount of air and sending it through the body in the right way to feed and nourish every cell with the oxygen it needs to create and continue to be in the flow. This discipline of effective breathing is a spiritual exercise as well as a physical one.

This picture of the whole person does not stop with the body. Far from it. In fact, Ayurveda was never limited to the state of the human body. Its original purpose was to encourage flow and health in the body in order that a human body could strive successfully toward spiritual attainment. Health was the vital step toward becoming holy. That does not mean, however, that ill people cannot reach spiritual attainment. In fact, many of the great swamis and spiritual teachers were afflicted with illnesses and painful conditions. However, they were able to demonstrate that it is entirely possible to become holy, to achieve great spiritual awakenings, even in frail flesh. However, they were unusual. It is probably truer for most people that the better we feel, the more we can push ourselves to spiritual attainment.

The great Rishis taught that our bodies are holy vessels and that we need to keep them well. This is similar to the Christian teaching that our bodies are temples. Both traditions

21

teach that this temple of flesh should be maintained as a place where holiness can reside. This is much in line with the great Tibetan Mahayana Buddhist teaching that human incarnation is rare and that we should not waste this opportunity. Whether it is rare or not, it is easy to see that it is a pity if we choose to subject our bodies to living conditions and habits that break them down and make us ill. We can see from this belief that many great spiritual traditions merely confirm that if we are to live as aware and awakening spiritual beings, we need to acknowledge our bodies as sacred. Ayurvedic teachings also confirm this point of view. We were meant to be whole and to be the best person we can possibly be.

All aspects of Ayurveda try to give us the opportunity to achieve this by enabling us to find and, when necessary, to restore lost harmony whenever it occurs. Deepak Chopra teaches that it is merely a by-product that we have the capacity to attain total wellness. This would be the difference between seeing an Ayurvedic practitioner and your local HMO doctor. One would see your wholeness as attainable, the other would focus on your symptoms without asking why you would have such symptoms.

3

Five Elements,
Three Doshas,
and More

Ayurveda takes all its references from the natural world around us and from the profound meditations of the Rishis from whom its teachings came. The Rishis lived in continuous states of higher consciousness and meditation, and from their deep mystical experiences they understood that the true nature of the world is energy. From this pure energy, which is not a measurable scientific force but a philosophical concept of consciousness, come the Five Elements that make up the material world we inhabit.

We find references to the Five Elements in three major medical systems: medieval European medical thought, traditional Chinese medicine, and Ayurvedic medicine. They tend to be interpreted differently, but they are clearly connected. We may assume from this that the ideas spread far and that the essential truthfulness of the Rishis' perceptions was apparent to others.

The term *Five Elements,* as interpreted by the Ayurvedic system, includes the elements of ether, air, fire, water, and earth. Harder to understand for most of us westerners is that each term does not really describe a fixed thing. It really describes processes, how things work, and how they are in relationship to each other. So, for example, the term *water* is not limited to what we know as water. It includes the idea of flow, of nourishment, of energy, of flow within ourselves and our material bodies—within our cells, within our consciousness, and within our spirit. The Five Elements is a whole concept that includes all these possible meanings. Everything in the material world is made up of the Five Elements in different proportions. The principle of "as above, so below" certainly applies here. The tradition of Ayurveda assumes that our bodies should reflect the nature of the universe and the way energy works in us.

THE FIVE ELEMENTS

Ether

Sometimes also translated as space, ether refers to both inner and outer space. Its outer form is the mind and consciousness, while inside the body ether can be found in the cavities, such as the mouth, abdomen, digestive tract, thorax, and lungs. In some of these, we can see how the concept connects with the structures of breathing. Some Ayurvedic experts also consider that it includes the idea of the spaces within the cells of our body as well as unlimited consciousness. It also corresponds to the sense of hearing, and relates to the ears. Its qualities are light and expansiveness.

Air

This is connected with the idea of the air we breathe, and nerve and sensory impulses. In its workings in the body, it includes muscle reflexes, the beating of the heart, the action of the lungs, the digestive processes, and the central nervous system. It corresponds to the sense of touch and relates to the skin. Its qualities are coldness, roughness, and dryness.

Fire

This is what results from the friction of air, and we find it in every process of the body that is thought to contain or need the action of heat. It is in the digestive system—think of the burning of indigestion, the body's metabolism, the body temperature—and is connected with the eyes and with intelligence. Hindu tradition thinks of eyes as showing the fire of the soul, and of intelligence as being a kind of mental fire. These are certainly metaphors that we are familiar with in the West. Fire corresponds to the sense of vision. Its related qualities are heat, clarity, and movement.

Water

We have already considered the concept of water, so we need only add that it is present in the saliva, the membranes, blood, and cells. It corresponds to the sense of taste and is related to the tongue. Its qualities are liquidity and soft oiliness.

Earth

This is a metaphor for the whole world of solid matter, and traditional Hindu wisdom considers that what we see and think of as solid matter is actually crystallized consciousness. Earth is connected with hair, skin, and nails, as well as with the structural helpers that literally hold us together—bones, tendons, ligaments, cartilage, and muscles. It corresponds to the sense of smell and to the nose. Its qualities are solidity, stability, slowness, and immobility.

From this, you can probably begin to see that the Five Elements are indeed complex and yet common sense. Remember that the first teachings of Ayurveda that came to us in the *Rig Veda* were in the form of poetry, and this has certainly influenced the way sages have continued to think of and explore their knowledge of health and healing. It still is as much an art form as it is a science.

So every different process creates an energy form of its own, and the teachings of Ayurveda state that the Five Elements combine to create three different energy forms, known in Sanskrit as the three doshas or Tridosha. The energies of the Tridosha are found only in living matter. It is the varied workings of the Tridosha that manifest themselves as our body, our flow patterns, our spiritual being, and also as imbalance, or the causes of our diseases. It is because of this that dosha means in Sanskrit "that which darkens or causes to decay."

Each dosha is made up of two of the Five Elements, which shape its characteristics. Ether and air create the air principle called *vata;* in Sanskrit this means "wind or the cause of movement." Fire and water combine to create the fire principle called *pitta;* in Sanskrit this means "which digests things." Earth and water combine to create the water principle known as *kapha;* in Sanskrit this means "which unifies." The three doshas—vata, pitta, and kapha—are known as the Tridosha.

THE TRIDOSHA

The concept of the Tridosha also occurs in Tibetan medicine and in European medicine. Its form and function may vary, but this way of describing how energy works in the body to create everything material is a common approach found in several early medicine systems.

We are born with our genetic and our karmic Tridosha in place. The particular dosha balance of our two parents creates our predominant dosha. This gives us our temperament, body type, propensity for particular illnesses, manifestations of imbalance, and so on. This is known as our basic constitution, a concept that Ayurveda also shares with homeopathy. Our whole life will be involved with being a constitutional type. We seldom change into a different constitutional type, unless other doshas are present that emerge more strongly at later ages. Therefore, if a person is born disabled, this might be a karmic manifestation, if it is not genetic. It would not be wise to assume that this means the person deserves to be born disabled because of a bad deed. Great spiritual teachers warn us that we have no idea how to judge another human being's karma. Karma is merely a consequence, or sometimes a choice. It is not a punishment. If you stick your finger in a flame, the karmic result will be that you get burned.

27

This does not mean the flame punished you. It is a result merely of sticking your finger in a flame. It might be that a profoundly spiritual person chose the difficulty of such a life to bring help and enlightenment to others.

BODY TYPES

Classically, Ayurvedic body types are clearly aligned to one of the Tridosha or to a classic combination of two of them. It is quite rare that a person manifests the qualities of all three doshas, although it can certainly happen. In Ayurveda, body type includes a picture of a person's mental, emotional, and spiritual character as well as the physical body.

Vata

A typical vata might be either very short or very tall, but with a slim body and light bone structure. This type of person will tend to be slender and will find it hard to gain weight, but a vata imbalance—due to poor eating habits—might challenge this belief. Vatas are darker than average and don't burn easily in the sun. Because they are cold types, they love warm climates and plenty of sunlight. Their eyes tend to be gray, dark blue, violet, or deep brown and it is not unusual for vatas to have two eyes of a different color. Vatas are high-energy people, restless, always on the go, and therefore prone to nervous exhaustion. They love vigorous exercise—aerobics, running—but should be encouraged instead to do yoga or tai chi, which is much more suitable for their body type. They are full of ideas, love new challenges, and are always ready for action. This is an excellent quality—however, they should take care to nurture themselves with times of rest, meditation, and withdrawal from the world. Otherwise, they become permanently exhausted, tired, and irritable and prone to states of anxiety and depression—this can be a sign of adrenal fatigue.

Expressive and outspoken, these types can be real movers and shakers with unusual vision and creativity. Without discipline though, they may be unfocused and unable to make their vision a reality. Healthwise, vata people might experience any of the following: skin problems, typically dry, irritated skin. Lacking oil in the skin, vatas may wrinkle early. Hair can be a real problem as well—dry, coarse, and dull, often with dandruff. Teeth have a tendency to be easily damaged, often with receding gums. Eating habits can be variable with this type but must be regular to keep a vata happy. Vatas do not do well with fasting and should be encouraged to avoid it. Constipation can also be a problem, but it can be controlled by good eating habits. They are light sleepers, often with insomnia and a tendency to wake in the night and be unable to go back to sleep. Vatas may suffer from emaciation and a sense of cold or bloating. Under stress, they can experience sensory disorientation, incoherence, and vertigo. Arthritis is one of the results of vata stress. They also fall prey to diseases of the nervous system, wandering aches and pains, and various intestinal afflictions. Vata energy becomes more dominant in old age—thus, the strokes and dementias of old age. Its season is fall; its times are sunrise and sunset.

29

Pitta

Pitta types are strong, active, and precise people who have no problem stating their case and making their wishes known. They are average in weight and build, with fair skin (compared with others of their race or ethnic type) subject to sensitivities and blemishes. They feel hot in almost any season and they have thin, fine hair, inclined to be oily. Their eyes are light in color, usually hazel, green, or light blue, and are easy to become inflamed. Their teeth are regular size, with gums easily inflamed or infected. They like their food and get grouchy when it is late or lacking. Their bowels work well and they sleep well, too. If they wake, they get back to sleep easily. They do badly in hot climates and poorly in difficult situations where their hot tempers might flare up. Fortunately, they have a good sense of humor and their sharp intelligence and facile tongue usually get them out of trouble. Their health problems are likely to be digestive, due to the fact that they live on nervous energy. They are usually overdrawn and can easily become ill. They may have liver trouble, burning sensations in the body, with fever, inflammations, or a sense of too much heat. They get herpes, eczema, and rashes easily and suffer from ulcers and irritable bowel syndrome or ulcerative colitis. They are also prone to blood diseases, fevers, infections, inflammations, and skin diseases. Since these are typical type A personalities, they may well end up with chronic fatigue, as well as liver ailments. Pitta energy rules transformation and adulthood. Its times are noon and midnight; its seasons are late spring and summer.

Kapha

Kapha people have the biggest builds of the three major types of doshas. They range from medium to large, or even very large. It is easy for them to gain weight and hard to lose it. Often, they have wonderful skin—smooth and moist. Typically, they have brown or black, wavy, strong-looking hair. Their eyes are peaceful and clear. They often have large, white, healthy teeth. Their elimination habits are good and without problems. They eat well—sometimes too well, hence their weight gain around the waist and hips. They can be sluggish and don't like exercise. They cope well with any climate, sleep well, but may wake up groggy. They have equable, often gentle, emotional attitudes. They often speak slowly and carefully, not wishing to rush into anything sudden. Kaphas give others a sense of reliability and strength without force. They are loving and well-grounded people. They have great fortitude and courage, and people love to be around them because they make others feel secure and appreciated. When they do get ill, they tend to suffer from lung and respiratory problems. Digestive troubles can include nausea and an inability to digest food well. Breathing problems, mucus production, yeast infections, and congestion are the kapha ailments. They also get water retention and blockages and may have a tendency to depression due to their discomfort with their own negative feelings. They may also accumulate too much weight, become lethargic and heavy, and sleep too much. When this happens, they need to be goaded and disciplined.

31

These are the three pure types of dosha and probably you recognize yourself in one of them. However, you may also feel that you have characteristics from another type, and you are probably right. Most people actually are two-dosha types.

Vata–Pitta

These people usually have the vata build and temperament—slender, fast—but use little nervous energy. This gives them more stamina and a keener intelligence. Pitta brings useful balance to vata.

Pitta–Vata

These people tend to have the pitta build—medium, sometimes gaining weight in middle age, but not too much. Their systems are not delicately balanced, and they like to forge ahead when faced with a challenge.

Pitta–Kapha

This type combines the kapha build with the pitta drive, which may overwhelm the naturally easygoing temperament of kapha. When kapha bulk has anger and negativity displayed, there may be a lot of pitta exhibited there. This type can achieve a lot. Large athletes are pitta-kaphas.

Kapha–Pitta

The difference between this and the previous two-dosha type is found in the rounder, fatter, softer appearance of this one. This type also takes a less aggressive stance toward life.

Vata–Kapha

This type pulls together two very different types and you'll recognize such a person by a vata build—slim, even skinny—allied
to a kapha's easygoing attitude. The two-dosha alliance may
show in kapha's lack of neurosis but with the occasional vata-
like outbreak of nervous stress.

If you are a two-dosha type, remember that your needs and per-
sonality may change as you age and your other dosha either
comes into play more strongly or recedes. The doshas are only
guidelines to help you identify your possible areas of concern so
that you can catch yourself before any manifestation of imbalance actually turns into a disease.

In the course of human life, we experience the dominance
of the Tridosha at various times. Kapha dominates in childhood
from birth to fourteen years; fourteen to twenty-seven years are
the pitta-kapha years; pitta rules in adulthood from twenty-seven
to forty-two years of age; forty-two to fifty-six are the vata–pitta
years; vata dominate from age fifty-six to seventy-seven; and
vata-kapha years are from seventy-seven to the end of one's life.
These time periods mean that the relevant dosha type should be
nurtured in order to maintain its natural balance.

Vata is nourished by light, warm, and moist climates, and
is most balanced when following gentle routines and listening to
gentle, harmonious sounds. Pitta does best with peaceful, cool
climates and enjoys wholesome, tasty, and calming foods while
carrying out restful, gentle meditative activities in beautiful sur-
roundings. Kapha people need to get moving and get busy, live
in a warm, dry climate, and eat small quantities of spicy foods.

33

They need to get to work in the kitchen, take care of the house, and get good exercise to keep that somnolent kapha energy on the move.

BALANCING YOUR DOSHA

There are four important ways to help yourself find this ideal balance—through diet, exercise, daily lifestyle, and seasonal routine.

Vata Balance

Vata is restored by routine. Easily exhausted, often overwrought, vata needs habit, rest, relaxation, good sleep, warmth, good food, plenty of fresh water to drink, and a regular sesame oil massage.

Here are your magical restoratives:

- Learn to meditate.
- Live in warm rooms.
- Eat well-balanced meals at regular times, concentrating on salty, sour, and sweet tastes and warm foods with great texture, all cooked with butter. These bring balance to vata, whereas bitter, astringent, or very pungent tastes cause imbalance. Think hearty home-cooked soups, homemade bread, slow casseroles, and fruit pies, eaten in a relaxed atmosphere. Vata does well with grain, dairy, a great breakfast, herbal teas, gentle spicy foods, and sweet fruits.
- Massage your body every morning with sesame oil.

- Take a long warm bath or shower in the morning before meditation.
- No violent entertainment at night.
- Surround yourself with bright colors.
- No alcohol, coffee, or nicotine.

Pitta Balance

In order to stay cool and learn how to relax, you need some moderation in your life. You love nature's beauty, so take the time to be with it at least once a day. Cut out your stimulants and work on balancing your active life with your relaxed life.

- Take it easy. Don't drive yourself. While balancing yourself, resolve to let go for a while. Really, the world will manage without you. If you are an angry, driven workaholic, watch out, you pitta. Make saving yourself a conscious effort.
- Let yourself wind down by creating a genuinely quiet evening for yourself.
- Learn to meditate.
- Keep cool. Bedroom below seventy degrees, no long hot baths.
- Drink cool, sweet drinks like apple juice.
- Eat right for your pitta nature. Include salads and vegetables, cold cereal, vegetarian food (yes, we know you don't want to—that's why it is especially good for you, pitta), high-carbohydrate foods, and Japanese and Chinese foods in your diet. Avoid pickles and other

sour foods, and don't eat Mexican, Indian, or fast foods. Avoid all sour, pungent, and salty tastes while you are trying to reach balance, and instead make sure you eat foods with sweet, bitter, or astringent tastes.

- Gradually reduce your food intake.
- No artificial stimulants.
- Walk at sunset, gaze at the moon, stroll by the lake—all great pitta-soothers.

Kapha Balance

Kaphas, on the other hand, need a little stimulation and regular exercise, not to mention weight control.

- Get out of your boring routine and bring a little variety into your life. Take a vacation in a far-away place or meet people in an interesting setting, and you'll feel like a new person.
- Eat the way you should, moving toward light foods with a minimum amount of butter, oil, and sugar in them. Eat hot food instead of cold, adding some bitter or spicy taste to every meal. Favor extra-hot Indian curries or chili-rich food. Cut back on candy, eat raw fruits and vegetables but no deep-fried anything, and watch those salad dressings. You find balance best with pungent, bitter, and astringent tastes, and you should avoid sweet, salty, and sour tastes.
- Stay warm.
- Don't get damp.

- Do a dry massage on your body, using a dry loofah and no oil, taking long, quick strokes.
- Drink some warm fluids daily, but not too much.
- Exercise regularly.

TRIDOSHA SEASONS

There are particular times of the day, seasons of the year, and times in a life when the various Tridosha are predominate. Kapha time is after dawn and after dusk. This can be when people suffering kapha conditions—mucus excess, for example—experience a worsening of their condition. The answer to this is to drink a mildly spicy tea and to avoid cold drinks and cheese, both of which increase mucus conditions. Kapha season is winter and early spring, with cold, damp, and foggy weather that requires kapha people to eat plenty of spicy food to keep in balance.

Pitta time is mid-afternoon and then again from 11 P.M. until around 2 A.M. Pitta disturbances, such as gall-bladder or liver conditions, may manifest themselves at such times. Sunrise and sunset, plus the hour just before each, is vata time. This is when meditation works most powerfully and when the human spirit is most in touch with the divine. It is also when people with vata disturbances feel them, awakening at 3 A.M. and being unable to get back to sleep due to worry. Autumn with its dry, cold, windy weather is the vata time of the year when vata people must be especially careful to look after themselves, stay in balance, and keep warm. Pitta people are most affected by the hot, humid season of late spring and early summer when they must be careful to eat cooling foods.

According to classical Ayurveda, there are actually six seasons to the year, with every two months being a season. It is at the changing of each season that there is the highest risk of falling ill, and each dosha type has a particular time at which to be especially careful to try to maintain balance.

Vata risk times are around mid-September and mid-November when vata people are encouraged to be patient and to eat vata-nurturing foods; kapha risk times are mid-January and mid-March when kaphas should be firm and disciplined about their food and live stoically; pitta risk times are mid-May and mid-July when pitta types have to be observant of their diet and attentive to their balance.

FOOD FOR YOUR DOSHA

Since the food we eat is a vital part of how we find balance, this section fully explores the variety of foods that best suit each of the Tridosha.

Vata types do best with well-cooked rice and oats. Fresh vegetables should be cooked for vatas and could include asparagus, beets, carrots, garlic, onions, radishes, and sweet potatoes. Members of the cabbage family should be steamed and added to soups and casseroles. Avoid fresh salads since vata does not do well with them. Ripe fruits like banana, cherries, grapefruit, mango, papaya, peaches, pears, pineapples, plum, and all citrus fruit are fine. No dried fruits. Vata does well with meat, but make it organic and preferably chicken. Fish is also excellent for vata types; they also cope well with dairy products. Nuts and seeds should be consumed in moderation—they help ground vata.

Pitta folks do best with a vegetarian diet in which moderation is observed in everything—not too hot, not too cold, not too spicy, sour, or salty. Steamed or stir-fried vegetables are good, and raw vegetables should only be consumed if the pitta digestive system is able to cope. Sweet and bitter vegetables are fine, but avoid tomatoes, radishes, garlic, and peppers. Choose from asparagus, beets, all cabbage family members, cucumbers, green beans, leafy greens of any kind, peas, potatoes, squash, sweet potatoes, and sprouts. Occasionally, onions can be eaten but they must be white or yellow. With fruits, sweet is good but sour is not. No papaya or bananas, but fresh figs, cherries, grapes, sweet apples, berries, fresh dates, melons, pears, and plums can all be eaten. Beware of sweet oranges and pineapples. No seafood for allergy-prone pittas; avoid most red meat, and stick with freshwater fish, chicken, turkey, and venison.

Pittas and all varieties of beans go well together, but avoid nuts. With dairy products, go for unsalted butter and cheese, cottage cheese, and unsweetened yogurt. Sweet tastes are soothing for pittas who can best use fructose, maple syrup, sucanat, and turbinado sugar. Honey and molasses should be avoided— they tend to be too heating for pittas. Pitta does well with a wide variety of grains—barley, rice, oats, wheat, or amaranth.

Fat-gathering kaphas should avoid greasy, fatty foods altogether and minimize sweet, sour, and salty tastes. In grains, kaphas can choose from buckwheat, millet, barley, rice, corn, muesli, dry oats, and polenta. Most vegetables are agreeable for kaphas; only sweet potatoes, squash, tomatoes, and cucumbers should be avoided. No sweet or sour fruits, but plenty of dried fruit is fine. Most meats are fine for kaphas, but they should

39

be roasted or broiled. A limited number of beans should be consumed—kaphas can pick from among aduki, black bean, garbanzo, lentils, Lima, navy, pinto, soy, and white beans. However, no nuts or seeds. Very few dairy products—minimal amounts of unsalted butter, low-fat cottage cheese, yogurt, and soy milk. Use raw honey in very small quantities. Use all spices, but avoid salt.

IMPORTANT AYURVEDIC TERMS

There are other important terms classified in Ayurveda that refer to significant subjects that play a part in creating the true balance of the body.

Agni

Agni (in Sanskrit "fire") is the energy that fires the digestive processes and guarantees all nutritional needs of the body are taken care of. It is also the energy that maintains the immune system. There are many factors that cause imbalance in the agni—eating wrongly, sleeping insufficiently, mental anxiety, ignoring the conditions for our dosha type, and so on. We maintain appropriate levels of agni by:

1. Eating the diet most suited to our dosha type.
2. Chewing our food completely.
3. Making sure our food is organic, unpolluted, and natural.
4. Taking bitter herbs that are good for the digestive processes.
5. Eating foods that are in season.

Ama

Ama is a waste product produced by ill-digested foods and toxicity that coats the inside of the colon. However, if it accumulates, it spreads to the blood vessels, capillaries, and arteries; therefore it may be considered to be the equivalent of mucus and cholesterol in Western medicine. It is regarded as one of the main factors in the course of developing an illness. It can be detected by an examination of the tongue. If the tongue is coated with a white substance, this is a sign of ama in the system.

Prakriti

Prakriti is the term for the basic constitution of each individual. Before any kind of Ayurvedic treatment can be started, the physician will establish what your basic constitution is since this will give the guidelines for needs, herbal remedies, and diet. From a detailed examination and questioning process, the doctor will find out which doshas predominate in you, and from that your prakriti becomes known.

Gunas

This term refers to the qualities of all organic and inorganic matter and describes linked pairs that balance each, like the yin and yang of traditional Chinese medicine. Contrary to what many westerners believe, these are not opposites. They are actually linked, balancing pairs. Think of the swing of the pendulum, rather than of opposing concepts.

The classical *gunas* include such pairs as hot and cold, soft and hard, oily and dry, heavy and light, sharp and dull, subtle and gross, smooth and rough, moving and still, transparent and opaque, solid and liquid. Each of the Tridosha relates to one or other of these gunas and foods, drinks, and herbs do as well. If dosha, guna, and food all have the same qualities, there will be imbalance. So, our task is to find the way to balance out the qualities and nature of each so that we pick balanced food and medicines for ourselves.

RASA: THE SIX TASTES

The term *rasa* or "taste" has a broad meaning. For example, taste can include the idea of the whole mechanism of taste, starting from the tongue, continuing its journey to the brain, stimulating responses, and beginning a chain reaction of process in the body. Rasa does mean taste, but it also includes such ideas as essence, vitality, juices, and sap. Its Sanskrit root also includes references to music and life. Rasa is necessary for the human being to become involved in eating. We can see this when elders lose their senses of taste and smell along with their appetites and interest in food. If food is only fuel, it does not really attract us. This is why we say in Ayurveda that rasa ignites agni, the digestive fire.

This is a metaphor for the rich and creative way in which food engages the human being. After all, as humans we cannot live on grass. We have a profoundly wide-ranging appetite for many kinds of foods and are capable of using and digesting a wide variety. Life really is a banquet for the average human being. The six classical rasa are sweet, salty, sour, pungent, bitter, and astringent.

Sweet

Sweet taste is found in sugars and starches, butter, milk, grains, sweet vegetables, and sweet fruit. Water, too, is thought of as being sweet, and it is this sweet taste that is considered to be the most dominant of all the rasa. This rasa builds the body and increases the kapha energy, which brings about calmness and soothes the mind. Sweet rasa is good for both vata and pitta people because it brings them the calm, strong qualities of kapha people. For kapha people, however, there must be limited use of this rasa since otherwise it brings about kapha imbalance. This rasa is associated with the elements of earth and water.

43

Salty

All kinds of salt are included here—sea, rock, table, and also seaweed. It helps the digestion and is considered soothing to body membranes, as well as being an occasional laxative. It is a stimulant and a cleanser and makes the kidneys function well. Most of the more watery vegetables are considered to be salty in taste. It is very good for vata people, but pitta and kapha should use it as little as possible. This rasa is associated with the elements of fire and water.

Sour

The rasa sour relieves thirst and is stimulating. It helps digestion, and it encourages the elimination of wastes from the body. It is found in such foods as yogurt, buttermilk, lemons, vinegar, and pickles. Also many fruit—such as strawberries—are considered to be sour as well as sweet. Vata types do very well with this taste. Sour is grounding and warming for vata, but kaphas need to keep their sour intake down, while pittas may react with a burning in the stomach or intestines.

Pungent

This rasa is found mainly in spices such as black pepper, chili, cayenne, asafoetida, garlic, ginger, and mustard, as well as in all essential oils. It is considered to be drying and stimulating. It increases body metabolism and acts as a decongestant. It is useful for all dosha types. Vatas find the pungent rasa helpful, but both pitta and kapha types should use it moderately. People with pitta conditions—inflammations or rashes—should forego pungent tastes. This rasa is associated with the elements of fire and air.

Bitter

This rasa is found in dark-green leafy vegetables, coffee, neem oil, turmeric, aloe vera, and in many herbs. The taste is detoxifying and restorative of function. It is good for the liver and helps heal skin ailments. It is a digestive aid. It is diuretic and therefore reduces body weight. Both kapha and pitta benefit from the bitter rasa, but vata people should largely avoid it or use it only in moderation. It is associated with the elements of ether and air.

Astringent

This drying, tonifying rasa should be used medicinally and in moderation. It helps heal excess discharges, such as diarrhea, sweating, bleeding, and others. It is found in beans, unripe bananas, persimmons, pomegranates, and cranberries. It also includes herbs such as witch hazel and raspberry leaves. It is also found in many teas, especially herbal teas with medicinal uses that are high in tannin. It is good for kaphas and pittas, drying them up and bringing more balance to them, but vatas should use it only in very small quantities. It is associated with the elements of earth and air.

VIPAKA

The process of appreciating food does not stop with rasa. There is a postdigestive result of eating foods that is called *vipaka*; this is a stage in which the original six rasa are synthesized into three tastes. Sweet stays sweet but salty becomes sweet. Pungent stays pungent but bitter and astringent both become pungent. Sour is still sour.

There is more to using food well than just cooking and eating, especially in the wisdom of Ayurveda. There is the injunction to eat foods in season and grown locally, or at least grown in a climate similar to the one where you live. There is also an attitude that involves being gracious and being grateful. In traditional Indian society, a small offering of the food is made to the fire itself as a sacred thank you to the divine universe. You may not have a fire to do this with, but you can offer your thanks in the same spirit of gratitude.

Ayurveda has other guidelines for harmonious relationship to food. They include:

- Not sleeping immediately after a meal, especially if you are overweight.
- Allowing a few hours to elapse between dinner and retiring for the night.
- Walking gently after meals to encourage good digestion of your food.
- Always sitting down to eat.
- Chewing your food properly.
- Being meditative in your eating.

4

Body Type
and Imbalance

In Western allopathic medicine, we pay no attention to body type as a way of recognizing our temperament, the conditions we typically manifest in our illnesses, or how we may best care for ourselves. The standard assumption of Western medicine is that we must all be stereotypes of exactly the same human body and emotional being. This patently absurd assumption is only found in modern Western allopathic medicine. No other working system of medicine in the world assumes this, from traditional Chinese medicine to homeopathy. In fact, recognizing our type is one of the major ways in which we begin to plan for our own needs as human beings. Ayurveda understands that there are a variety of human types, each with special needs, special capacities, and special ways of manifesting imbalance and ultimately disease.

Of course, people vary infinitely from each other, but we do find there are certain patterns that may rightly be assumed to indicate certain recurrent types. With its three-thousand-year history, Ayurveda has had the time frame within which to draw up a valid pattern of these types and what we might call an energy style that operates in the body at all its levels. In the Middle Ages in Europe, concepts of this kind were often used to describe human beings, and they were known as "humors." These work in balance with each other and, when they are imbalanced, they will seek to regain their original balance. Their imbalance comes about because the dosha is aggravated by adverse conditions. Its energy becomes excessive and this excess energy brings about disease.

Such imbalance creates what we would recognize as symptoms of illness, and an Ayurvedic physician would recognize from these symptoms which part of the energy system of the Tridosha needs expert adjustment.

CORRESPONDING PROCESSES OF THE TRIDOSHA

Vata Processes

These processes are believed to be air, wind, and space, and they control the basic life force in a body. They are centered in the colon and control the digestive processes. They are also involved with breathing and circulation. Vata is connected with certain qualities—dryness, cold, changeability. It governs the emotions of fear, nervousness, and the qualities of spirituality and higher consciousness. Areas of the body that are most connected with vata are the colon and also the skin, bones, and nervous system.

Pitta Processes

These are thought of as fire and water and can include any aspect of body health that could be imagined as needing fire or water. This could be anything from the fire for living to the fire of digestive processes. Emotionally, pitta is our energy for life, the power of enthusiasm and enjoyment, and it may also emerge as anger and criticism. It is thought to control intestines, blood, eyes, and sweat and sebaceous glands.

49

Kapha Processes

These are considered to be water and earth related and are the ways in which our bodies are grounded in the flesh. Emotionally, kapha refers to love, compassion, forgiveness, and could also refer to self-pity and greed. Physically, kapha controls energy storage, joints, and body fluids.

When we are in balance, we live and act according to our basic constitution, called prakriti in Sanskrit. Prakriti refers to the balance of the three dosha energies within us, even though we may be predominantly one type. When modern life and our own bad habits put us out of balance, we are likely to manifest the illnesses typical of our dosha type. This is another very important departure from the typical Western way of thinking about diseases. Mainstream medicine assumes that germs, bacteria, viruses, body systems gone awry, and accidents are the reason for most of our ill health. Ayurveda—and traditional Chinese medicine and homeopathy, for that matter—assumes that we live imbalanced lives that open up the possibilities for illness. Germs, bacteria, and viruses are always around—the fact that we are sometimes caught by them has more to do with the state of our immune system. The state of our immune system is closely linked to our state of balance and harmony.

There are ways in which we already know that the assumptions we make about illness in the West are wrong. We think about germs, bacteria, virus, genetics, and yet we have other intuitions about what really allows illnesses to manifest themselves. There are traditionally three causes of imbalance of the doshas as discussed in the next section. They are misuse of the mind and body, over- or understimulated sensory organs, and disregard of the natural rhythms of the world.

CAUSES OF IMBALANCE

Misuse of the mind and body includes a wide variety of actions such as holding back the natural urges of the body as expressed in coughing, sneezing, and elimination. Overstimulated sexual activity, inappropriate behavior, and failing to follow therapy are all misuses of mind and body. It also includes every kind of reprehensible social behavior—drunkenness, immodesty, being in company with degraded people, giving free rein to character defects, and generally behaving badly. Misuse of the senses includes: staring too long at bright objects, seeing frightening or disgusting things, or not using the eyes at all; listening to harsh, noisy or unpleasant sounds, or listening to disturbing messages about unpleasant things; smelling ugly or unpleasant smells; eating the wrong things in the wrong amounts; excessive bathing, massage, or use of oils on the body. There are appropriate actions, behaviors, and routines for the days of the years and for the years of our lives, and to breach these will lead to sickness and imbalance.

The following pages outline the typical picture of imbalances to be found in each type. However, these symptoms are not necessarily linked to only one type of dosha. They could also arise out of other imbalanced doshas, which can imbalance each other and change the general functioning of the whole.

51

Vata Imbalance

Vata types, for example, are prone to nervous system diseases and intestinal disorders; both of these problems are typical of the person who lives much of his or her life on a mental level and may be suppressing a great deal of emotional baggage. Such people frequently have headaches, general weakness, and may suffer from deterioration of the nerve tissue of the body and atrophy. Vata imbalance also produces speech defects, sore throats, tonsillitis, earache, and stomach and intestinal problems. The earliest sign of imbalance is likely to appear in the colon and can include cramps, genitourinary disorders, menstrual and prostate problems, lower-back pain, and muscle spasms. High blood pressure, blood circulation problems, and heart murmurs, along with stress-related nervous disorders, are likely to abound in people with imbalanced vata.

Mental and emotional disorders are not uncommon when vata becomes imbalanced. You will find that many people who have chronic fatigue syndrome, fibromyalgia, or lupus are very likely to be vata types, as are those who have multiple chemical sensitivities. Since these are not robust people, they are likely to have easily compromised immune systems. They often find it very hard to sleep well, or they wake early and are unable to get back to sleep. Thus, they often deplete the reserves of energy that help them face the day. Because of this slight fragility of the immune system, vata people are somewhat sensitive to medication, may have poor responses to medicines, and often have allergic reactions. They need lower doses of medicines than the other dosha types, along with careful monitoring. Vata people should carefully document their experiences with medicines, herbs, and remedies so they can be alert for adverse reactions.

Vata types also have a particular response to symptoms, and from those symptoms we can also read their imbalances and their needs. Here are typical vata problems:

- General coldness in the body.
- Intestinal gas and burping.
- Joints make cracking sounds.
- When in pain, they typically have severe, throbbing, intense pains.
- When vatas are sick with a fever, they are thirsty, anxious, and restless but do not really have very high body temperatures. Because of their type, they may actually be more ill with a lower temperature than the other dosha types.

- When they have a cough, it tends to be dry and without much mucus, but they often find it hard to breathe.
- Their sore throat feels rough and hot with a painful squeezing sensation in the esophagus.
- Since they are often constipated and may have difficult bowel movements, their stool is small and dry.
- Skin imbalance shows as dry, rough, and flaky skin that must be treated regularly with oil.

Vata illnesses come on fast and are worse at dawn and dusk. Fall and winter are their worst seasons for getting ill, and weather conditions of windiness, cold, and dryness increase the severity. Vata needs to avoid the following foods when ill: dry foods, beans, cold foods, raw foods, carbonated drinks, and caffeine. Vatas should seek herbal remedies among the following herbs: codonopsis, American ginseng, dong quai, angelica, marshmallow root, aloe vera juice, ashwagandha, slippery elm, and licorice root. To calm those vata nerves, try one of the following: basil, biota seeds, valerian, jujube dates, oat straw. Other herbs that make life more gentle for easily disturbed vata types are orange peel, fresh ginger, fennel, hawthorn, sassafras, sarsaparilla, lemon grass, and rosehips. Many of these strengthen the functioning of the body—ginger is good for the stomach and digestive system, hawthorn is a great heart helper, and rose hips are bursting with vitamin C, which will strengthen the immune system. A massage oil that is great for vata is sesame oil mixed equally with almond oil. Add a few drops of the essential oils of lavender and rose geranium—both are great emotional supporters and are calming and soothing to the whole being.

Pitta Imbalance

When pitta types get sick—which is not often since they have pretty good resistance when they stay in balance with life—they are likely to have illnesses that fall within the following range: fevers, infections, inflammations, ulcers and colitis, blood diseases, rashes, red itching skin disease, and various inflammatory conditions. These are diseases of overheated or out-of-control pitta energy.

They often suffer from imbalances of the liver and gall bladder and experience hyperacidity in the body. Digestive disturbances of many kinds appear in people with imbalanced pitta, as do problems with the blood itself. Production of red blood cells, the balance of blood and jaundice, anemia and other blood disorders such as leukemia, are found in pitta people. Eye problems and skin problems, including skin cancer, are signs of pitta imbalance.

The typical ways in which pitta types manifest illness and imbalance include the following:

- Overheating in various parts of the body.
- Bleeding, production of pus, inflammation, and various rashes.
- Pain that tends to be of medium intensity but often with a burning quality to it.
- Fevers that include high temperatures accompanied by thirst, sweating, and even delirium.
- A cough that is usually accompanied by a sense of heat and which produces a lot of phlegm, often yellow or green in color.

- Sore throats that feel inflamed and burning.
- Digestive problems, such as sour burps with heartburn.
- Uncontrolled diarrhea with watery, yellowish stools that leave a burning sensation.
- Urinary problems include color change to deep yellow or even a reddish shade with increased frequency and burning sensations.

When pittas get ill, it usually comes on slowly with a fever, and they feel worst at noon and midnight. Summer and late spring are the most vulnerable times for sickness to come on a pitta, especially when it is hot and humid. Pittas should always avoid hot and spicy foods along with salty or sour foods. Pittas should give up meat and acidic foods along with tomatoes and caffeine. Visitors to sick pittas should know in advance that their emotions will include irritation, impatience, anger, and frustration. That may be partly due to their disturbed sleep patterns—bad dreams, night sweats, fitful sleep.

There are a range of herbal teas especially suited to pitta, and they include alfalfa, catnip, chickweed, cleavers, mint, nettles, and raspberry. It would be fine to use an herbal tincture—which is probably much easier to find—and add it to hot water.

To calm your pitta fire, use the following herbs and essential oils: avena sativa, chamomile, kava, lavender, Melissa, oat straw, passion flower, and skullcap. Do *not* take essential oils internally; just enjoy aromatherapy from them.

Pittas typically suffer from liver imbalances, which is why they need to cool down by having toxins removed from the body

55

through special herbs. These include barberry bark, burdock root, dandelion, milk thistle, red clover, and yellow dock. These can be combined or you can simply pick one. Even if you are well, pitta, think about using these herbs from time to time to keep yourself in balance. Always drink plenty of water when taking any of these herbs because they cleanse toxins out of your body, and good elimination is essential. Other good tools to help with typical pitta conditions of inflammation and infection are the following: echinacea, goldenseal, Oregon graperoot, and usnea.

Kapha Imbalance

Kapha types do not become ill easily. They are robust, balanced people who are pretty stable in life. Their illnesses tend to arise from their ability to be still—sometimes too still—and to carry a lot of body bulk. Thus, they are most likely to be found suffering from mucus diseases, respiratory problems, water retention, depression, and emotional blockage. When kaphas are sick, they are prone to feeling pain that is heavy, dull, and constant, often with a low-grade fever that persists for a long time and a great feeling of heaviness and lassitude.

Their typical symptoms when ill include many of the following:

- A cough that is very congested and filled with mucus.
- A sore throat that feels full and swollen.
- Digestion that becomes slow and heavy, leaving the feeling that food is lying undigested in the stomach for a long time.

- A stool that is enlarged and often full of mucus.
- Urination that is infrequent and pale-looking.
- Edema that is present in the skin.

Kaphas become ill slowly and then stay that way for quite a while, feeling worse at mid-morning and mid-evening. Dampness and cold aggravate sickness, which is most likely to come to kaphas in late winter and early spring. They need to avoid dairy products, salty and sweet foods, cold drinks, fried food, and caffeine. When ill, kaphas will feel sorry for themselves and often become depressed, apathetic, lethargic, and dull, and will sleep for long periods at a time. The following herbs will help kapha people with cleansing: barberry, bayberry bark, burdock, dandelion, hops, juniper, milk thistle, Oregon grape, and turmeric. To help with their mucus conditions, kaphas can use elecampane, garlic, ginger, grindelia, hyssop, licorice, marshmallow root, and thyme. For their depression, kaphas can use chamomile, lavender, and lemon balm.

5

The Great
Medicine Garden

As with all traditional systems of healing, Ayurveda makes great use of medicinal plants. Many of the greatest allies are those we in the West identify as herbs, spices, and aromatic roots we normally use in the kitchen. Of course, it was through the daily use of such plants that people learned of their helpful and healing qualities. An important part of Ayurveda is that it encourages us to look at food and drink not only as something to fill ourselves with but as a tool for health and healing.

This chapter begins with a useful list of the most common healing herbs, spices, and oils, which are all easily available to most people living in the West. Following this is a more specialized list of important herbs and medicinals that can be obtained from herbal resources listed in the resources section.

COMMON HEALING PLANTS

Since every culture develops the medicinal solutions for its most common ailments, we should not be surprised to find that many of the medicinal herbs and spices of India are used to treat intestinal and digestive problems, as well as fevers and skin conditions. These form the majority of the ailments and afflictions of everyday life in India. Remember, it is not unusual in India for plagues and epidemics to occur. The most common of these are cholera, typhoid, meningitis, hepatitis, malaria, and yellow fever. This is why Ayurveda has effective treatments for many of these conditions.

Aloe Vera

Originating in tropical Africa, this plant was brought to India by the Chinese in trading expeditions. The plant can be used in a dried form as a bitter herb, or the gel can be scraped out and used to cool inflammations, heal burns, and reduce infection in wounds or cuts. It will help lower the temperature in cases of sunburn, too. In India, a traditional way of using this plant is as a fermented aloe. The gel is fermented with honey and spices and then used as a tonic. It is good in cases of anemia, poor digestion, and liver disorder.

Aloe has a great power to bring balance back to the body. It is used to help women who suffer from menstrual cramps. Take one or two teaspoons of the fresh gel and add a pinch of black pepper. Two teaspoons of fresh gel can be taken daily to help liver problems, ulcers, and colitis. Aloe can be used internally as a douche in cases of vaginitis by adding two tablespoons of fresh aloe to one quart of warm water.

Holy Basil

The basil plant, known in Sanskrit as *tulsi,* is often planted in temple courtyards in India, hence its popular name Holy Basil. Often, Indian families keep a small Holy Basil plant at home and honor it in their rituals of worship. It can be used fresh as an herb in cooking and also in its essential oil form, when it is used as a massage oil diluted in a carrier oil such as sweet almond oil. Holy basil is used as a heart medicine, and modern research indicates its helpfulness in lowering blood pressure and in lowering blood sugar levels in people with diabetes. This undoubtedly has connections with the finding that Italians—who eat fats and drink wine but also eat basil and garlic together as pesto—have a heart attack rate much lower than we think they should, considering their rich diet.

Basil also has strong anti-inflammatory properties, pain-reducing capability, and fever-reducing powers. The leaves are chewed and eaten for treatment of many small ailments. One teaspoon of the leaves, juiced, plus a teaspoon of ginger juice and a pinch of pepper will help healing from fever, colds, or indigestion. A traditional Ayurvedic recipe is to mix basil leaves, black pepper, ginger, and honey, and to eat this to prevent infection and to reduce high fevers. In Ayurveda, it is believed that half a teaspoon of fresh basil juice can be given to babies to control fevers, and that this juice can also be used to fight ear infections by putting drops into the affected ear. Basil has great powers to help reduce stress and is considered to be an adaptogen in helping people deal with and transcend stress without it taking a physical toll. One more use: If you've been bitten or stung, squeeze some basil leaves and then rub them against the wound. It will instantly begin to soothe and heal.

Cardamom

Chewing the seed helps indigestion and stomach spasms. Added to food, cardamom makes it more digestible, which is one reason why it is often found in sweet milk desserts. Be aware that the white cardamom pods found in this country are not the healing cardamoms used in India. In India, cardamoms do not have a white hull, but are brown and used when the interior seeds are blackish brown and therefore at their medicinal best. Chewing cardamom seeds keeps your breath sweet and your teeth healthy. It is also helpful for digestive problems and upset stomachs, and therefore it is good medicine for travelers to carry with them. It helps sore throats and is considered to be good for singers. Powdered cardamom is not a good replacement for the seeds and will probably be too old to be medicinally effective.

Castor Oil

The seeds of the castor oil plant are highly toxic, but this toxicity does not pass into the extracted oil. Traditionally in India, women massage castor oil onto their breasts to help stimulate the flow of milk after giving birth. Also, herbal poultices are made of the seeds to help swollen joints. Used internally, the oil is a strong laxative. Used as a compress over the liver, it is said to help serious liver ailments.

Cayenne Pepper

Cayenne pepper has many powerful healing properties, some of which we are now becoming familiar with in the West. For example, far from disrupting the digestive process, cayenne actually stimulates the stomach to work efficiently and helps heal ulcers by promoting good digestion. It promotes sweating and attacks colds and flu through its antibacterial powers. It can be gargled to help with throat problems and laryngitis. Rubbing on an ointment containing cayenne helps ease the pain of arthritis, rheumatism, and shingles. Since this is a powerful agent, it must be used with caution. There are safe ways to use it. You can make tea from it by adding a teaspoon of the powder to a cup of boiling water, then taking one tablespoon of this infusion and diluting it further in another cup of water. Then sip as needed when you have a cold, chill, cool hands or feet, or are suffering from shock or depression. You can also throw a teaspoonful of the powder into a hot bath when you feel you are coming down with a cold. It will heat you up and burn out the cold.

63

Cinnamon

Cinnamon is regarded as a tonic herb that promotes circulation. In India, it is most often used as a tea and it relieves fever, headaches, and chills. It has antiviral and antibiotic powers in fighting infection. The essential oil has powerful pain-relieving qualities when massaged into the skin. If you make a tea from the bark, it helps diarrhea and kidney complaints. Tea made from twigs of the cinnamon plant is great for colds and stomach chills. Pregnant women must *not* use cinnamon, especially cinnamon essential oil, since it is a uterine stimulant.

Cloves

In cases of nausea or vomiting, especially when caused by food poisoning, put one or two drops—no more—of the essential oil on a sugar cube and eat it. If you do not have the essential oil, make a tea from the clove buds and drink it for the same results. Its use in cases of toothache is well-known in the West; it also has powerful antiviral and antibiotic qualities and is frequently found in powdered form in Ayurvedic toothpaste. The essential oil, mixed with a carrier oil such as sweet almond oil, can be rubbed on the skin in cases of fungal infections. It is also a local antiseptic.

Coriander

Coriander is found almost all over the world and has a long recorded history of use dating from the earliest medicinal text in the world, about 1500 B.C. The upper leaves are known as cilantro and the little round seeds as coriander. The plant also produces an essential oil, which should not be taken internally. Long regarded in Europe as an aphrodisiac, it is used as a tea for intestinal disturbances of various kinds in Indian herbal repertoire. It helps flatulence, bloating, cramps, and intestinal cramps. It is considered very useful for reducing fevers caused by excessive heat and promotes good brain and nerve function. Chewing the seeds also sweetens the breath. Ten drops in two tablespoons of carrier oil can be massaged into swollen joints, arthritic areas, and places where fluid has accumulated. Breathing coriander essential oil helps the nervous system, boosts the immune system, and helps migraines and neuralgia.

Cumin

The seeds are used as a spice in cooking and are considered to help the digestive system. Cumin relieves bloating and flatulence, and helps the entire gut to relax. In India, cumin is regarded as being helpful in cases of insomnia and is used to treat colds and fevers. Mothers who are breast-feeding eat the seeds to help with milk production. Ground-up cumin seeds are mixed with onion juice to make a paste that is applied to scorpion stings to relieve the pain and swelling.

Fennel

Fennel seeds are those little seeds that you find in most good Indian restaurants. Take a pinch and chew them as an aid to digestion. A tea made from the seeds helps to promote breast-feeding and soothes a baby's colic because the active principles from the fennel are absorbed in the mother's milk. However, pregnant women should be very cautious about using this as it is a uterine stimulant. Tea made from the seeds also soothes the digestive system of anyone suffering from flatulence, indigestion, or colic. You can also use this tea as a mouthwash and a gargle for gum disorders, loose teeth, laryngitis, and sore throats.

65

Flax Seeds

Flax seeds have so many uses that the Emperor Charlemagne passed a law requiring citizens to eat the seeds to maintain good health. The ripe seeds help a congested chest to clear through productive coughing. Making a tea from the seeds will help a sore throat. You may also add honey and lemon to this brew. Eating the ripe seeds helps constipation, but it is important to also drink a large amount of water.

If you have boils, abscesses, or ulcers, you can crush the seeds and press them against the infected area. People suffering from eczema, rheumatoid arthritis, and atherosclerosis should eat one or two teaspoons of the crushed seed every day. The whole plant can be used to make a tea that relieves constipation, liver congestion, and rheumatic pain. Be cautious about using flax since the seeds contain traces of prussic acid. Don't be too alarmed—apple seeds contain traces of cyanide—but don't exceed suggested doses, either. *Never* use the linseed oil sold in art stores for consumption or internal use.

Garlic

Garlic is a major ingredient in Indian cooking, and it helps keep the digestive tract healthy, cleanses the blood, and reduces inflammations and infections. In the case of ear infections, traditional Ayurvedic healers insert a whole garlic clove and pour in oil, sealing the ear overnight with a wad of cotton wool to allow the garlic and oil to do their healing work. Mashed and crushed garlic is also used as a poultice on wounds, boils, and inflammations. Garlic is regarded as one of the most versatile of healers because it has such a wide range of applications. Most people benefit from eating at least two cloves of garlic a day. It prevents arthritis and helps maintain normal blood pressure. Recent studies confirm that it lowers cholesterol and blood pressure, and that it may be a powerful preventive in heart attacks. Ayurvedic tradition suggests that garlic can be chopped up and used on wounds and indeed it can—but be aware that fresh chopped garlic placed on the skin will strip the surface away! Only if you were in serious danger of, for example, dying from septic wounds should you even consider such action. Otherwise, never place raw garlic next to the skin. Instead, use a poultice or compress.

Ginger

This root, which is such a kitchen favorite, is a very powerful nontoxic medicinal plant with many useful properties. It heats up the body and drives out fevers and chills. It helps in respiratory conditions and colds. It supports liver and kidney function, and treats nausea, sickness, vomiting, and morning sickness. It is a great help in digestive processes, and it has powerful antiseptic qualities that make it useful when taken internally in cases of food poisoning. To treat nausea, an ounce of fresh gingerroot can be chopped up and simmered in two cupfuls of water until the liquid is reduced by half. Then it may be sipped throughout the day. In France, doctors prescribe one or two drops of essential oil of ginger on a sugar lump to be eaten as a help for flatulence, fevers, and to stimulate the appetite. Add a few drops of essential oil to two tablespoons of carrier oil and massage into places that suffer rheumatic pain and areas where bone injuries ache. Ginger is safe to use in moderation only in early pregnancy.

67

Lemon

Lemon is a fruit native to India. It is considered to be useful in staving off colds and, taken in warm water each morning, is a great liver helper. So much so that one of its traditional uses is as a treatment for hepatitis.

Nutmeg

The kernel of the nutmeg has been mainly used for digestive help when a person is suffering from nausea, vomiting, diarrhea, food poisoning, and indigestion. The kernel can be made into a tea and drunk three times a day as a digestive treatment. This works better if it is also mixed with ginger and licorice root. In modern Western medicine, nutmeg has been used successfully as a treatment for Crohn's disease. The essential oil can be added—ten drops only—to two tablespoons of carrier oil and used to massage painful muscles that have been overexerted by physical activity. It also helps in cases of rheumatism and arthritis when massaged around painful joints. *Never* use the essential oil without dilution and be very careful about ingesting nutmeg. Large doses produce convulsions and palpitations.

In France, doctors recommend putting three to five drops of nutmeg essential oil on a sugar lump for nausea, gastroenteritis, chronic diarrhea, and indigestion.

Pomegranate

Parts of the pomegranate are used in a traditional mixture to treat dysentery. Its rind and fruit parts can also be processed to treat tapeworm infestation, but this must be done by an expert since the bitter alkaloids in the pomegranate can be extremely toxic. Do not even think about trying this at home.

Turmeric

This root is related to the gingerroot and shares some of the same qualities. In India, turmeric is a traditional remedy for jaundice and liver trouble, and recent research has confirmed its powers to restore liver function. It is a strong anti-inflammatory, more so than the drug hydrocortisone, and is traditionally used for arthritis and rheumatic pains. It is also regarded as helpful in treating asthma and eczema. To treat athlete's foot, grind up some turmeric root and mix it with a small amount of calendula ointment, then rub the mixture on. It makes a very effective treatment.

ESSENTIAL OILS

Essential oils are also an important part of the Ayurvedic repertoire of healing helpers, as well as being used for ritual and religious purposes. They are wonderful healing and emotionally helpful substances with a long history of use by humankind. However, they must be used with respect. They are very powerful and contain many active constituents, some of which can harm you. They can be fatal if swallowed. Unless you are under the treatment of a skilled aromatherapist, *never* ingest any essential oil and be careful which ones you use directly on the skin. Only lavender and rose geranium are safe for almost anyone to use directly on the skin. Otherwise, either use them in a diffuser or add a few drops to your bath and soak in the perfumed water.

Never use artificial or chemical oils for aromatherapy purposes. Be aware that unless a product says it is pure essential oil or 100 percent essential oil, it probably is not. Never use perfume oils for aromatherapy purposes. Remember that when you breathe in or have a massage with essential oils, you are absorbing them into your body. Never do this with anything other than pure essential oils and, even then, be careful that you know which ones are good for you. A much fuller introduction to essential oils and how to use them in your everyday life will be found in chapter 7, "Using Healing Oils."

Essential Oils and the Tridosha

Each of the Tridosha has essential oils that are considered to be especially supportive for one of the three types. For vata types, the most helpful essential oils are angelica, basil, cardamom, cinnamon, frankincense, jasmine, lavender, orange, rose geranium, and sandalwood. These help stressed-out, out-there vatas to relax and become grounded and warmed. Pitta types do very well with the cooling, calming, and meditative essential oils of fennel, jasmine, lavender, lemon grass, orange, peppermint, rose geranium, sandalwood, and vetiver. Kaphas respond well to the awakening and energizing essential oils of cedar, cinnamon, frankincense, juniper, rosemary, sage, and thyme.

MEDICINAL HERBS IN AYURVEDA

Arjuna

Known as *Terminalia arjuna*, arjuna is one of the mainstays of Ayurvedic herbal medicine. Its bark has been used medicinally in India for over three thousand years. Confirmed by modern pharmacological research, it is well known for being good for the heart, with the first official prescription being written for this use by the seventh-century A.D. physician Vagbhata. It is a cardiac tonic, treating poor cardiovascular circulation with some success. It is best used for ischemic heart disease, and it treats angina successfully. It also lowers cholesterol. Because of the aid it provides to those with cardiovascular problems, this plant bark also treats edema successfully.

Traditionally in Ayurveda, a juice extracted from the leaves of the tree also treats earache. The bark can be used as a decoction to treat diarrhea and dysentery. In powder form, the bark is used in cases of asthma. It is also useful in cases of snakebite or scorpion stings. Ayurvedic physicians also used arjuna to treat patients who are suffering from excess in any of the Tridosha. This plant bark brings the Tridosha into balance again.

Asafoetida

Also known as devil's dung, asafoetida is grown mainly in the Indian subcontinent and west Asia, and produces a gum that has a distinctive smell.

This gum is harvested in summer from the root of four-year-old plants. It exudes from cuts made in the one giant taproot, which is the main body of the plant underground. The seventh-century *Charaka Samhita* says that this is the best remedy for intestinal gas and bloating. It was for this use that it also became known in Europe during the Middle Ages, probably after being brought back from Asia by crusaders returning from the Holy Wars. The volatile oil in asafoetida is effective as an expectorant, clearing the lungs of gathered mucus. This makes it useful in the treatment of bronchitis, bronchial asthma, and other respiratory problems. It is also used as a blood thinner and to lower blood pressure. *Never* use this with young children.

Ashwagandha

Known as *Withania somnifera*, ashwagandha is a tonic herb and all parts are used—roots, leaves, and berries. Some herbalists call it the Indian ginseng because it has the power to help all the systems of the body. It is an adaptogen, which means it stimulates or sedates body organ function as needed. It has constituents that are anticancerous and act as natural anti-inflammatory steroid hormones. This was confirmed in laboratory studies carried out in the 1970s, during which cancer cell experiments showed the growth-inhibiting capabilities of this plant. It is the leaves that have this capacity in greatest measure. Its use in Ayurveda is to strengthen the whole system; mind, body, and spirit. It balances the system by reducing kapha and vata. It helps people to relax, sleep well, and be less stressed. The root is powdered and taken as a drink for its tonic action. People recovering from long illnesses chew fresh or dried berries to increase their powers of recovery. Since the plant is known to have the ability to be a restorative, it can help repair damage of long-term stress; it could be explored usefully by anyone dealing with chronic fatigue syndrome.

Calamus

Known also as sweet flag and, in Hindi, *bacc*, this plant originated in India but is now found all over the world and is a very important part of the Ayurvedic herbal repertoire. In Ayurvedic tradition, the calamus root is thought of as a rejuvenator of the brain and nervous system, and it is taken in powdered form made from the root of the plant. It also aids the digestive system by stimulating appetite while calming indigestion, colic, and relieving intestinal gas. The Ayurvedic herb is called *Acorus calamus* and is *not* the same variety as the American sweet flag, which is *Acorus calamus americanus*. The Ayurvedic herb is banned in some countries, an indicator that you must use it with caution, preferably under the guidance of a skilled herbalist. Do *not* use it for more than one month.

Cardiospermum

Found all over the tropical world, this plant, also called the balloon vine, is a climbing plant of which roots, leaves, and seeds all have medicinal applications. In India, the root is used to bring on delayed menstruation and to relieve arthritis and backache. Applied locally, the leaves stimulate circulation and are often crushed and used as a compress on swollen, aching joints. The seeds are dried, crushed, and swallowed in water to help arthritis. The whole plant has sedative qualities. This plant should be avoided by pregnant women.

Chiretta

Native to India, this is a powerfully bitter herb and is therefore considered to be very suitable for quenching the fire of pitta conditions. Because of its bitterness, it is considered a great tonic, especially for the liver. It is also known for stimulating appetite, helping stomach pain, and reducing fevers of all kinds. Research in India shows that this plant has antimalarial qualities and protects against tuberculosis. Chiretta is a great aid for weak stomachs, especially when the stomach manifests such symptoms as nausea, indigestion, and bloating. It is taken as an infusion in tiny doses to help the whole digestive system. It also helps in cases of worms.

Elecampane

This is a legendary plant, getting its Latin name *Inula helenium* from Helen of Troy who was said to have set off for Troy holding this plant. It is the root of the plant that is used, both in dried and fresh form, and its main use is in respiratory problems, being effective and safe for people of all ages and states of health. The root has antiseptic qualities, and, as a good expectorant, it helps clear the lungs in respiratory illnesses. It can be used for bronchitis and asthma, especially in their chronic forms, and it both soothes the lungs and gently stimulates the coughing reflex to encourage the coughing up of mucus. In India, the root is also considered as a great help for the digestive system, helping the appetite and relieving indigestion. In the past, it has been used to treat tuberculosis, and its restorative tonic action is as valuable as its ability to fight infection.

Galangal

Known as *Alpinia officinarum*, this is an Indian member of the ginger family, used as a medicinal root that will help stomach upsets, inflammation, and respiratory conditions. Research from China has shown that it has an antibacterial action against a number of pathogens, including anthrax. Other research shows it is effective against intestinal candida. In India, it is either used as a tea, sipped slowly, or dried and ground up to be used as a powder, taken in tea or water. It is regarded as being very soothing for the nerves and effective in treating stomach pain, dyspepsia, rheumatoid arthritis (because of its heating qualities), and, for the same reason, good for fever. It was introduced to Europe in about the tenth century by Arab traders and later by Hildegard of Bingen, a famous herbalist and mystic, who referred to it as the spice of life.

Gotu Kola

Also known as Indian pennywort, gotu kola is known as an herb that can help brain and nervous function and is becoming well known in the West among those who wish to preserve or improve their memory function. Traditionally, in India, it has been used extensively to treat skin conditions, including leprosy, skin ulcers, and sores. For this use, a paste is made from powdered dried leaves, which are then mixed with water, and the resulting mixture is applied to the site of skin disturbances, such as patches of eczema. Typically it is used as a salad or vegetable in India or, dried, the leaves may be ground into a powder and drunk in a tea or applied as a paste to the skin.

Known as a rejuvenator, in India it is also considered to be a remedy for infertility and a tonic for poor digestion and rheumatism. For these purposes, it is usually made into a tea that is drunk several times a day. Fresh leaves are fed to children to help fight dysentery, and the plant is also thought to be good for asthma, fevers, and bronchitis. In the West, it is now being used for memory problems and rheumatism.

Licorice

This has been a part of the herbal traditions of both the West and the East for thousands of years. This powerfully sweet herb is regarded as having many healing virtues, including the power to help gums and teeth remain healthy. The most commonly used part of the herb is the dried root, which is often used as a natural toothbrush by Indians. Laboratory testing of licorice has revealed that it has exceptional antiplaque qualities. Used in powder form, it is taken to relieve sore throats and can be sprinkled on wounds to prevent infection. In laboratory research studies, it has been found that this plant has a powerful anti-inflammatory and antiarthritic effect, as well as being very effective in helping people with chronic hepatitis and liver cirrhosis. This makes it a possible ally in the current silent epidemic of hepatitis C in the United States. You can use it safely and easily for mouth and tongue ulcers and infected gums by applying a dab of the tincture. You may also consider buying it powdered and making your own toothpaste of myrrh and licorice powder. You will never have gingivitis if you do this. If you want to impart a more familiar flavor to this paste, add a few drops of peppermint oil.

Shatavari

Also known as *Asparagus racemosus*, this is regarded as one of the great tonics for improving blood and body fluids. It is the root which is used, either as a tea or powdered, and taken in a drink. This is especially good for strengthening the female reproductive system, and it promotes the production of milk in nursing mothers. It is also thought of as promoting fertility and having a certain capacity to enable the development of spiritual awareness and compassion.

Varuna

Known as *barun* in Hindi, this tree grows throughout India and has a three-thousand-year-old documentation of use for a variety of problems. Its key actions, now confirmed by modern scientific research, are to act as a diuretic and to prevent kidney stones. Varuna works by increasing bladder function and by reducing production of the oxalates in the body that are responsible for the formation of kidney stones. It also seems to slow the actual rate at which stone-forming elements are deposited in the kidneys.

Extensive research has been undertaken in India in recent decades that has confirmed varuna as an effective treatment for urinary tract infections and bladder problems caused by enlarged prostate glands. Varuna's effectiveness for these problems was first documented in the eighth century B.C., and by the end of the first millennium it was accepted as the best treatment for most kidney problems. A tea made from the dried bark is taken at the rate of one cup three times a day to prevent the formation of stones. To treat urinary infections, the powdered bark is taken in water once a day. There are also other traditional uses for varuna. It is good for all weakened vata and kapha conditions and is used to treat bronchitis, asthma, and skin problems. The bark is also used to treat fevers, gastritis, and vomiting. The leaves can be bruised and mixed with vinegar to make a relieving poultice for inflamed joints.

Vervain

Verbena officinalis has been used as a sacred plant in many different traditions, from the druids to the Romans and in India where it is one of the great helpers of women. The arial parts of the plant can be used in a tea during labor to stimulate contractions and later to help the flow of milk. It is a good nerve tonic, helpful for nervous tension and anxiety. It stimulates the liver and urinary systems to cleanse out toxins from the body. This makes it very useful in the treatment of hepatitis. It is also helpful for migraine headaches, maybe because of its ability to clean out toxins. The plant can be crushed up to make a poultice to take care of wounds and skin sores. Chewed, it will help gum infections. Vervain is also one of Dr. Edward Bach's original twelve homeopathic flower remedies, the one which he recommends for mental stress and overexertion. It is a great helper for those recovering from a long illness.

6

Coping with Common Ailments

ARTHRITIS

This very common ailment is thought to result from a complex interaction of causes, from poor eating habits to emotional, environmental, and temperature issues. Ayurveda takes a holistic view of arthritis and treats it on the many levels at which it has its roots. It is most likely to be found in a vata type due to excess vata, but it could also be found in other types in whom vata excess energy has accumulated. The first step would be to cool the vata excess through diet. Good things to add to the diet would be sweet fresh fruit of all kinds; most dairy products; cooked vegetables; most natural sugars like honey, maple syrup, and molasses; seafood; eggs; small amounts of nuts; any spices; herbal teas like basil, chamomile, fresh ginger, or licorice. No wheat or yeast products shall be eaten. Note that wine would never be included in a good Ayurvedic diet, nor would any other alcohol.

It takes time to ease vata excess, so give yourself at least six months on this careful diet to see a real and permanent improvement in your arthritis. Also, remember to nurture yourself and face up to any undealt-with emotions (especially suppressed anger and resentment), as they are important factors in arthritis. Begin peaceful exercises such as tai chi or yoga and take up meditation. A traditional treatment for localized pain is to make a poultice of lobelia, cayenne, and cardamom powder, mixed with honey and clove oil to form a paste that you rub on the affected area and leave for about thirty minutes. Wash it off and you should feel the pain, heat, and congestion has left the joint.

COLD/FLU

Vata-type cold and flu symptoms would include the following:

- Dry cough
- Dry nose or throat
- Mucus clear and not much of it
- Insomnia
- Chills
- Fever, possibly intermittent
- Emotionally upset, restless, and perhaps fearful

If any of these symptoms describes you, you need to be heated and hydrated. Take a good hot bath with a handful of ginger powder thrown in the water. This will drive up your temperature and will often burn out a cold or fever before it really takes hold. Drink warming spice teas such as ginger, cardamom, and cinnamon. A heating pad might be comforting for you. If you are eating, keep it simple and light. Take some herbs to boost your immune system—echinacea or licorice root. For your dry nasal passage, dab a spot of sesame oil at the base of each nostril.

Pitta-type colds and flu look like this:

- High fever
- Burning
- Yellow or green mucus
- Sore throat
- Agitation

If you can eat, keep it light and simple. Avoid meat and dairy while you're ill. Herbs that will cool you down are burdock, elder flower, peppermint, yarrow, lemon balm, and mint. You can take some of these in a tea. Echinacea and goldenseal should be taken every two hours until you feel better. For your sore throat, put three drops of tea tree oil in warm water for a gargle. You could also use your echinacea and goldenseal in this way too.

Kapha-style symptoms include:

- Low-grade fever
- Loss of appetite
- Excess mucus
- Excess saliva
- Mucus in stool or urine
- Lethargy

If you wish to eat, keep it very light—no meat, cheese, or bread. Any bitter herbs may help—dandelion or burdock, for example, taken in a tea or tincture. To make yourself stronger, sip ginger tea, adding honey if you wish, throughout the day. Take echinacea and goldenseal every two hours to support your immune system and work against inflammation and bacterial infection. If you get the chills, take a hot bath with powdered ginger in it.

COUGH

A vata-style cough is dry and there is little or no phlegm. If there is a coughing spasm, it produces pain in the heart, chest, or throat. It is helpful to use herbs that will soften and ease this condition by allowing mucus to be more easily expelled. The herbs that do this include licorice root, comfrey root, and marshmallow root. You can also make teas from cardamom and ginger and either drink them separately or brew everything up in one tea. You can ease tightness in the chest by gently rubbing niaouli essential oil on the chest and lung area.

With a pitta cough comes green, yellow, or blood-streaked phlegm. There may be a burning feeling in the lungs, as well as a fever and thirst. Use those powerful antibiotic herbs —echinacea and goldenseal—and repeat every hour until you begin to feel improvement. To soften and help removal of the phlegm, use licorice root and marshmallow root. Angelica root and leaves are also expectorants and antiseptics and can be used as a tea or tincture.

If you have a cough with lots of phlegm and chest congestion, this is a kapha disorder whether or not you are a kapha. Learn from good kaphas and cut out cold drinks, fruit juice, and heavy foods like cheese, milk, dairy, white sugar, and anything fried. Ginger tea will help. It will warm you and keep your system working against the infection. Using eucalyptus essential oil will help to keep your air passages open. You can either add a few drops of eucalyptus oil to sesame oil and massage it on your chest, or you can burn it in an aromatherapy pot.

SORE THROAT

A vata sore throat feels dry and scratchy, maybe with some hoarseness. You won't experience much pain on swallowing or a feeling of congestion. Classic treatment for this is grandmother's time-tested recipe—lemon and honey in hot water, sipped. You can also either burn frankincense resin or burn essential oil in an aromatherapy pot.

83

A pitta sore throat feels very painful, like strep throat. Use echinacea, goldenseal, and usnea hourly. Lemon and honey will help the pain, and you can add tea tree drops to hot water and gargle.

A kapha sore throat feels full and swollen. A lot of mucus forming in the throat needs warming herbs such as the following: sage, bayberry, turmeric, garlic, or cloves. Garlic is a powerful antiseptic that will help any infection; you can also use sage tea as a gargle.

FATIGUE

In Ayurveda, this is a large category that includes nervousness, exhaustion, anxiety, and insomnia, as well as generalized fatigue, including what is now called chronic fatigue syndrome and fibromyalgia. This is considered to be a lifestyle problem, in which the individual has lived without reference to the real needs of the body and its essential pattern of balance. Ayurveda says, and our own bodies agree, that we cannot live in balance-bankruptcy. If we disregard the needs of our type and ignore the energy levels of our bodies, we have to reach the point of collapse. In modern times, when many people and life itself is lived out of balance, this has become an epidemic.

Here are the basic causes of this kind of imbalance:

- Poor eating patterns, including irregular meals composed of the wrong kinds of food.
- Too much caffeine.
- Poor exercise habits, either excessive exercise or not enough exercise.
- Overexposure to electronic circuits.
- Overwork.
- Too much noise.
- Excessive sexual activity.

The beginning of healing starts with paying attention to the list of lifestyle imbalances. You cannot live an unbalanced life and find harmony in yourself or in your body.

Vata fatigue includes an inability to sleep combined with anxiety. Other signs of a vata imbalance include the following: a regular pattern of indigestion, suffering from phobias and general fearfulness, being spacy and unable to concentrate, eating binges, feelings of being unable to breathe properly, heart palpitations, an inability to concentrate, emotional emptiness, and nightmares.

Most of the solution is in your own hands. A good, steady routine that includes eating well and avoiding stimulants of all kinds will help. At night, before you go to bed, massage your feet with sweet almond or sesame oil to which you have added a few drops of lavender or rose geranium essential oil. Begin meditating morning and night, including chanting or saying affirmations. There are many herbs that are specifically useful for the symptoms of this imbalance. They include the following:

- For relaxation, oat straw or *Avena sativa.*
- For sleeping, valerian or hops.
- For general tonification, licorice root.
- For better vascular circulation throughout your whole body, gotu kola.
- For calming, soothing, and easing nervousness and tension, lavender essential oil used day and night in an aromatherapy pot.

85

Eat well and stimulate your poor digestion by adding mild spices to your food. Chew your food thoroughly and always make your meals peaceful, quiet times.

Pitta fatigue is usually caused by different problems, often wild emotions like rage, hate, and angry blaming of others. Overactive pitta emotions bring about many of the same problems that vata-fatigue types have, but with added heat, turmoil, and disturbance. These are exacerbated by the following:

- Being competitive.
- Running on ego.
- Eating the wrong foods that are overloaded with hot spices, fats, and hard-to-digest ingredients.

- Being a control freak.
- Watching too much violent entertainment.

You have to take yourself in hand if you don't want to continue on to the inevitable heart attack, stroke, or cancer that lies ahead. Start eating in a way that will be healthier for you— no excess spices, and cut down on both salty and sour tastes. Try strolling in the moonlight or beside a lake or the ocean. At night, massage your feet with coconut oil to which you have added a few drops of sandalwood oil. You can also touch one drop of sandalwood to your brow chakra or Third Eye, which will chill out your overactive mind. The following herbs will continue the process:

- Passion flower to relax you.
- Hops to help you sleep.
- Lemon balm to quiet your mind.
- Licorice root to fortify your system.

All of these herbs can be taken as a tincture or made into a tea.

Kapha fatigue: even kaphas get worn out. That big calm exterior may be housing an overanxious, exhausted mind that cannot rest. Many of the same Ayurvedic guidelines apply—live with a gentle routine; eat regularly but not too much; avoid dairy, meat, fried foods, and caffeine. Massage and exercise help, too.

Use the following calming herbs:

Hops, passion flower, chamomile.

There are no shortcuts in dealing with chronic fatigue or fibromyalgia. These conditions demand a complete change of life and, if you do not undertake it willingly, your energy level will force you to do so by bottoming out so that you must stop. As well as paying attention to the needs of your type, all sufferers from these conditions must address the following issues:

- Ask what is your real purpose in life and how you can support it.
- Undertake a disciplined meditation routine.
- Began a gentle exercise routine based on yoga to make you functional again.
- Be prepared to stick with these changes indefinitely.

87

CONSTIPATION

The colon is regarded as the site of vata energy and therefore constipation is always a sign of vata excess. Your bowel movements may indicate other excess energies as well though—dry stools being a sign of pitta excess, and stools with a lot of mucus showing kapha excess. Eating badly is the most common cause of constipation, followed by irregular lifestyle in general, and disregarding the natural urge for elimination when it occurs. The other major factor is drinking too little water. Change your diet to one suitable for your type; sleep at regular hours; nurture good elimination habits by trying to have a bowel movement at the same time every day, preferably early morning; and drink a glass of warm water before going to the bathroom to help things get going.

EMOTIONAL IMBALANCES

Since many illnesses begin in the energy system, they may manifest in your emotions before anywhere else. In fact, your emotions may well bring about an illness if you allow them to become excessive. Each type is especially prone to certain emotional imbalances.

- Vata emotional imbalance is likely to appear as nervousness, anxiety, fear, confusion, sadness, moodiness, and insecurity.
- Pitta emotional imbalance is likely to be anger, envy, fear of failure, frustration, hatred, jealousy, pridefulness, and spite.
- Kapha emotional imbalance is likely to be boredom, lack of compassion, greediness, obsessive behavior, carelessness, and lack of interest in anything.

88

For some reason, we in the West seem to consider that emotions merely happen to us, yet they are like any other aspect of our being. They respond to good management and the right lifestyle. If you become aware that your emotions are negative and are driving out the joy in your life, begin to take charge of them by reasserting a way of life that nurtures your type. Eat, rest, and honor your needs according to your type, and you will gradually find that your emotions begin to get back into good balance again. Becoming healthy in this way is as simple as it is in most other ways. The way in which we become ill may be complex, but the way in which we can become well is simple. It depends upon routine, sleep, rest, food, and living in accordance with the needs of our type. It may sound oversimple, but health solutions often are.

INDIGESTION

Most of us know why we get indigestion. We eat the wrong foods at the wrong times and in the wrong amounts. Ayurveda, being such a great system of true balance, suggests that the first step in dealing with digestive problems is to set that part of your regime right. In fact, the classic suggestion is that you stop eating for a while. Fasting for two days, drinking only water and fresh fruit juices, gives a great boost to your overworked digestive system. There are also a number of ways in which you can strengthen your system so it copes better, some of them involving the use of spices. If you have poor digestion and a weak stomach, cayenne pepper can enable your stomach to get back to its work. This is because, by Ayurvedic diagnosis, a weak stomach lacks the fire necessary to do its job. Sticking to bland or acidic foods, like milk, only makes the problem worse.

89

Here is a list of ways to improve your digestive system:

1. Drink fresh lemon juice in warm water three times a day.
2. Either chew a piece of fresh gingerroot with a pinch of salt five minutes before each meal or make a tea out of fresh gingerroot and sip this throughout the day. Both give your weak digestive system the fire it needs to get to work. Typical Western medical advice to stick to a bland diet only makes the problem worse.

A lack of spices means that there is nothing to spur the stomach into digesting food, no fire for the process.

3. Indian restaurants typically have small bowls of anise seeds available so that diners can take a handful to chew after their meals. This licorice-flavored spice helps the stomach to work better. You can buy it at most supermarkets in the spice section.

4. If you have flatulence or a burning in your stomach, drink plain club soda, and it will rebalance your system. Never take chalky indigestion pills since they do nothing to help rebalance your system.

5. When cooking, use all the digestion-friendly spices such as ginger, cumin, coriander, black pepper, and asafoetida. The first four are all available at your local supermarket, and asafoetida can be obtained from most Asian food markets.

6. Drink spicy tea during the day, using cinnamon, ginger, or cardamom as the spice.

To decide how to help yourself, you need first to figure out which dosha type your indigestion most resembles. For example, vata-type indigestion manifests typically as follows:

- Gas
- Bloating
- Constipation
- Insomnia
- Nervousness

It is very important for you to try to relax more and not eat when disturbed or emotionally upset. Don't eat on the run either. Instead, take regular meals in peaceful situations. Use spices and meditation to help yourself.

If, on the other hand, you have pitta-type indigestion, your symptoms will resemble the following:

- Heartburn
- Hyperacidity
- Diarrhea or loose stool
- Irritability
- Gas
- Localized burning when passing a stool
- Rash or redness of the skin

You should avoid spices and all acidic foods. Think instead of digestion-aiding herbs such as fennel, coriander, and mint. Also think about taking some bitter herbs, which are very good for settling pitta-style digestive problems. Dandelion would be great, along with Oregon grape root, and both are commonly available in tincture form from most health food stores. Young dandelion leaves make a wonderful bitter salad green, and you can always mix them in with sweeter salad items. Make a tea of coriander, cumin, or fennel. Although technically a spice, cumin is not considered a heating spice and so will help pitta-style indigestion. Drinking aloe juice on a regular basis will help cool down your overheated system nicely, too.

If you suffer from a kapha-style indigestion problem, you will have the following symptoms:

- Vomiting
- Mucus in throat after meals
- Desire to sleep after eating

91

You may be eating too many dairy products (including your favorite ice cream), too many fried foods, or maybe food that has been cooked in rancid fat. Get back to a more healthy diet, following the guidelines for the kapha type. The spices that will help you include cayenne, ginger, black pepper, cinnamon, cloves, and cardamom.

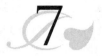

Using Healing Oils

Ayurveda makes great use of the rich bounty of nature and nowhere is this more apparent than in the use of oils, both regular oils and essential oils. This is a very powerful mode of healing and especially valuable in establishing that wonderful balance that is at the heart of a truly healthy life.

Among the oils used as a basis for whole-body massage are the following:

- *Sweet almond oil:* a rich but light oil, suitable for all skin types and nourishing for the skin. It leaves no greasy feeling on the skin and is easily absorbed so it can soften the skin and protect it against hot, dry climate conditions. It has no discernible scent.
- *Sesame oil:* usually associated with cooking in the West but greatly valued in Ayurvedic tradition as a massage

oil and regarded as one of the great therapeutic oils, especially for vata people. It has been used medicinally since the time of the pharaohs when it was made into ointments. It is warm, comforting, and grounding, as well as being rich. It is used in the special healing treatments of the Panchakarma.

- *Coconut oil:* thick and often solidified in anywhere other than the warmest climates. In India, of course, it is almost always found in liquid form. This powerfully protective oil gives the most natural sunscreen protection. Indians will often dress their hair with coconut oil because it keeps hair shining and healthy and does not let it dry out.

- *Neem:* neem oil comes from the seeds of the neem tree, a large evergreen native to India and virtually an entire medicine chest of its own. Every part of the neem tree has some special healing capacity. The bark is made into a tea for hemorrhoid treatment. The leaves are steeped to treat malaria and internal worms. The juice is expressed from the leaves to treat boils, ulcers, and eczema. The twigs are used for tooth-cleaning and treatment of gums. The oil is powerfully antiviral and antibacterial, and it is rubbed onto the head to prevent lice. It has also been traditionally used to treat leprosy. It is used as a massage oil when fever is present, and it brings down the body temperature. It has a fairly strong smell and most westerners are unlikely to enjoy its use as a massage oil.

Other oils that are not part of the Ayurvedic tradition but which you may well wish to use for an excellent carrier oil include the following:

- *Jojoba:* very rich and excellent for skin and hair health. It is usually quite expensive, so add only a small quantity to your main carrier oil to get the benefits of this enriching treat. If you have four ounces of massage oil, make one of them jojoba.
- *Avocado oil:* another of those wonderful skin treats to be added in moderation to your carrier oil.
- *Apricot kernel oil:* this has many of the good qualities of sweet almond oil and is a little lighter and silkier on the skin. It will blend nicely with any of the other carrier oils.
- *Grapeseed oil:* this greenish, light oil feeds the skin like apricot oil and sweet almond oil but is a little lighter on the skin.
- *Rose hip oil:* not often found but said to be one of the most restorative of oils for the face, probably due to its high vitamin C content. Add a little to your carrier oil.

Feel free to experiment with your blending until you find the mixture that is best for you. You are an individual so your needs will be individual, too. Mixing oils is more of an art than an exact science, and you can't do any harm with carrier oils, provided they are natural.

Do *not* use mineral oil under any circumstances since it carries petrochemical pollutants into your body. Also avoid all

95

products labeled vegetable oils, and be cautious about using peanut oil since much of what is commercially available is rancid and polluted. If you can get organically produced peanut oil, then you may use that. You can also use some of the more rare nut oils in moderation. These include walnut, kukui nut, and hazelnut. A wonderful skin oil is, of course, olive oil. Use extra virgin olive oil and blend it with others of your choice.

ESSENTIAL OILS

Essential oils give plants their aroma. Not every plant has an essential oil, and even those that do may not have much. Some of the richest and rarest oils come from plants that produce only a tiny amount. It takes one ton of rose petals to produce about ten ounces of rose oil.

Essential oils have powerful healing and therapeutic abilities, and they enter the body through the nose when we smell them and through the skin when they are used in massage. When we smell essential oils, the nasal cavity carries the molecules to the smell receptors in the brain. These then distribute messages throughout the limbic system that bring about responses throughout the body. When essential oils are used in a carrier oil, their molecular structure allows the healing essences to enter the bloodstream within an hour of being used in a massage. They should *only* be used in two ways: in massage oil and through breathing in the aroma. Most essential oils are *not* safe to take internally. A number should *not* even be inhaled. Avoid all the essential-oil multilevel marketing schemes. They are overpriced and overhyped and, in some cases, are encouraging positively dangerous practices, such as taking essential oils internally.

There are plenty of sources for essential oils, and several are listed in the resources section. These suppliers are reputed to have excellent, 100 percent pure oils that are first-class quality. Remember, if you buy expensive essential oils, they should be expensive. If you buy half an ounce of rose oil that costs less than $30, it is not pure rose; likewise for sandalwood, angelica, jasmine, gardenia, and myrrh. Excellent quality essential oils are produced by Nature's Alchemy, Tifferet, Starwest, and Aura Cacia.

Blending your own oils is easy and fun. When adding essential oils to a carrier, use only a few drops at a time for each ounce. For a strong-smelling oil, adding as few as four drops could be adequate. For a milder one, as many as ten drops might be suitable. Use your nose as your guide, since the strength of the aromatic oil has everything to do with its power.

97

Angelica

Angelica essential oil comes from the roots and rhizomes and the fruit and seeds of the plant. It has been used since ancient times, and its properties include strengthening the heart, stimulating the immune system, and increasing circulation. In aromatherapy, it helps make the skin beautiful and aids bronchitis and coughing. This oil has a tonic action on the whole body. It sets the lymphatic system to work and aids the cleansing out of toxins. It is very helpful after periods of extended illness. Used in massage across the abdomen, it helps ease colic and most digestive upsets. Rubbed on the chest, it helps bronchitis and other chest complaints. Put into bath water, it helps cystitis since it is antiseptic. Inhaled, it helps clear the lungs and improves breathing for people with asthma. It is also reputed to be helpful in increasing lung function in longtime smokers. It has the ability to restore feelings of balance and to relieve nervous exhaustion. These are reasons why it is a great oil for vata people.

Basil

98

Basil is called *tulsi* in Hindi and, since it is known for growing in temple courtyards, it is often known as Holy Basil. According to Indian tradition, it is sacred to the gods Krishna and Vishnu and therefore has protective spiritual qualities.

This is a stimulating oil, and it should be avoided in pregnancy. It can also be a dermal irritant for some people, so do a patch test on your skin first. Do not use it pure but dilute with massage oil. Used either as a massage oil or inhaled, it is employed for a wide variety of ailments in Ayurveda. Among them are bronchitis, coughs, colds, asthma, flu, and emphysema. Held under the nose, it revives people who have fainted. It is also considered to be an effective antidote to snakebite and scorpion stings. It is a nerve tonic and is naturally calming. Breathing it helps asthmatics and acts as both a mood elevator and a soothing agent. Used in massage and rubbed over the stomach, it relieves gastric spasms and eases nausea and dyspepsia. It imitates estrogen and is often used in massage when there are menstrual problems. It regulates the menstrual cycle. In childbirth, it helps bring about rapid expulsion of afterbirth. Made into a compress, it helps swollen breasts.

Basil strengthens the nervous system, calms hysteria, and eases depression. It is good for vata and kapha people.

Cardamom

This has been used in India for three thousand years, especially for lung disease, digestive upsets, fever, and urinary problems. Added to a carrier oil and massaged into the abdomen, this stimulates digestion and reduces gastric upsets such as heartburn, colic, and flatulence. Inhaling the aroma reduces nausea and encourages the flow of saliva. It is useful in easing coughs and helps with respiratory problems. It is uplifting and helps in cases of fatigue and weaknesses. It is for vata people.

Cedarwood

This oil comes from the Himalayan deodar cedar, and it has been traditionally used in the making of sacred incense for use in temples. It can be added to shampoo to help hair health and to fight dandruff, greasy hair, and hair loss. Added to a carrier oil, it is good for muscle aches and arthritis pain. Breathed in, it helps bronchitis, catarrh, and chest congestion and also has a drying effect on phlegm. Adding some drops to bath oil helps to reduce genitourinary problems and can soothe the burning of cystitis. It is also calming and soothing. It is *not* for pregnant women as it can cause abortions. It is for kapha types.

Cinnamon

Cinnamon is native to all the Indian subcontinent and is a tropical evergreen of which both the bark and the leaves are used for essential oil. The traditional use for this oil was making incense sticks for temple rituals, and it is said that it was associated with the mythical Phoenix. Cinnamon sticks, which most of us are familiar with, are taken from the inner bark of new shoots. Cinnamon oil is a powerful antiseptic, and the traditional use for cinnamon essential oil is to treat colds, flu, digestive and menstrual problems, rheumatism, kidney problems, and as a stimulating oil. It is very important that you *never* use cinnamon bark oil, which is a dermal toxin and mucous membrane irritant. *Always* be sure you are using cinnamon leaf oil. Added to shampoo, it is a treatment for scabies and lice. You can dab it on wasp stings to neutralize the poison and numb the pain. Added to a massage oil, it is a great helper with rheumatism and arthritis. It will help ease local congestion and will act as a pain reducer while also bringing better circulation to the area afflicted. It can also be massaged across the whole abdomen to help with menstrual dysfunction, intestinal spasms, and diarrhea. For colds and flu, soaking in a bath with a few drops of cinnamon leaf oil will drive out infection and get rid of congestion. Pregnant women should be careful since cinnamon leaf oil may bring on contractions. Cinnamon is for vata and kapha types.

100

Cloves

Another evergreen, the clove tree grows to forty feet and is found all over Asia where it has been cultivated in plantations for two thousand years. Use only the clove bud oil, not the leaf, but be aware that even the clove bud oil can cause dermal irritation in many people. As an essential oil, it can be used to treat athlete's foot and other fungal infections, and it can be used as an analgesic for tooth pain. In massage oil, it acts as an insect repellent and eases rheumatic and muscle pains. Breathed in directly or added to a hot bath, it aids breathing, eases asthma and congestion from colds or flu, and helps in bronchitis. As a stimulating and energizing oil, it is very suitable for kapha types.

Fennel

There are two kinds of fennel, sweet and bitter. Sweet is found only in cultivation but bitter grows wild. Although sweet fennel is regarded as safe to use on the skin, it is bitter fennel that is regarded as being the more powerful medicine and is the fennel used in Ayurveda. It must *not* be applied directly to the skin, however. Also, people with epilepsy and pregnant women should *avoid* using fennel. Its main uses are tonifying the liver, helping digestive problems, and dealing with obstructions of the liver, spleen, and gall bladder. It relieves gas, is antispasmodic, helps relieve stomachache, and is anti-inflammatory. The essential oil is made from sweet fennel and must be used externally. Added to massage oil it can be rubbed across the abdominal area to aid digestion and to relax the abdominal muscles.

Frankincense

Frankincense comes from a small shrub known as the olibanum and has been used in India, China, and the West in religious ritual.

In ancient Egypt, it was used in cosmetics, and medicinally it has been used for treatment of syphilis, rheumatism, respiratory diseases, urinary tract complaints, and skin diseases. The essential oil is made from the oleo gum resin, which comes from the plant. This can be added to the water in which you bathe your face to help diminish wrinkles and to nourish your skin. It has powerful healing properties for the nervous system and, inhaled, it is healing for the lungs. It has the property of making breathing slow and deep, which is why asthmatics can derive help from frankincense. This is also why its use is associated with sacred worship. That same capacity to help breathing is supportive of meditative and prayer states. A traditional belief about frankincense is that it protects the user from psychic attack and evil influences.

Geranium

Geranium essential oil comes from a plant known as rose geranium (*Pelargonium graveolens*), and its therapeutic uses include helping conditions such as dysentery, hemorrhoids, inflammation, excess menstrual bleeding, and many skin problems. It is one of the few essential oils gentle enough to use directly on the skin, although you should always conduct your own patch test to make sure you aren't one of the hypersensitive people whom it may affect. It can be used directly on bruises, acne, burns, cuts, and skin conditions like eczema and dermatitis. It helps in fighting lice and ringworm, and it acts as a mosquito repellent. Add it to a massage oil carrier, and you can rub it on areas afflicted by cellulitis and swollen and congested areas. It also helps edema and poor circulation. Rose geranium is also one of the greatest helpers for emotional states such as depression, anxiety, nervousness, and general stress and tension. If you know someone who gets anxious as evening comes on, try rose geranium on them.

Jasmine

Jasmine has many healing uses, and in its herbal form it has been a powerful helper in both Chinese and Western medicine. In China, the flowers are used to treat inflammatory conditions and serious liver ailments, while the root is used for pains of rheumatism, joints, and the head. The essential oil is among the most complex of all the oils, having over one hundred constituents. Its powerful aroma means that it must usually be used in very small quantities. It has a wide range of uses—from skin care, to muscle aches and pains, to respiratory diseases, to the genitourinary and the nervous systems. It can be mixed with a carrier oil and applied to the skin to help where it is dry or irritated. It will balance out greasy facial skin. Added to a massage oil, it will ease muscle aches, pains, and sprains, and you can also massage the abdomen to help uterine disorders, painful periods, and labor pains. Because of its power to stimulate the hormones, it should not be used by a pregnant woman until the hour of giving birth has approached. Then it will help the mother to deliver safely. It strengthens contractions and relieves pain at the same time. Breathing in the essential oil aroma helps soothe coughs, laryngitis, and catarrh. It also relieves spasms of the bronchi. One of the most powerful uses of jasmine is in helping the nervous system, especially in cases of depression, fatigue, and stress. It raises the spirits and brings back hope and optimism.

Lavender

This is the great mother oil of all the essential oils. It has many wonderful uses and it is gentle enough to be used directly on the skin of even a newborn. Since it has over one hundred constituents, it is laden with active ingredients to help and heal many ailments. Lavender can be used directly on the skin for many problems—abscesses, ulcers, boils, wounds, bites and infections, inflammation, and burns. It promotes the new growth of healthy skin and is effective against the wear and tear of aging upon the skin, especially facial skin. A drop can be put into the ear to cure earache or on the site of a snakebite, where it acts as an antivenom. It is powerful enough to fight gangrenous wounds and tropical ulcers. It reduces pain and nervous excitability, and its ability to help people sleep is very well documented at this point. One drop of oil on each temple will cure the average headache in ten minutes. Powerfully endowed with antibacterial capacity, it is also antiviral and fights throat and chest infections, even being considered helpful in fighting tuberculosis. Used as an insecticide, it keeps moths and other insects away. It makes the air pure to breathe. It treats psoriasis, ringworm, scabies, and spots. Added to shampoo, it will help cure dandruff. Used pure or added to a carrier, it helps a woman to expel afterbirth when rubbed on the lower back. Its greatest power in many ways is as an emotional helper. It is very effective in cases of depression and helps manic-depressives. It soothes hyperactive children, calms the old who suffer with dementia, and eases anger and resentment. It calms the mind enough that even insomniacs can sleep well when they have the aroma of lavender essential oil in the bedroom. With its many healing abilities, this oil is suitable for all the Tridosha types—vata, pitta, and kapha.

Lemongrass

Lemongrass, known in Hindi as *chumana pulu*, is actually a grass, though hard and woody in texture. It is native to India and found throughout most of Asia. Two varieties of grass yield this oil. Traditionally in Ayurveda, it has been used as a treatment for infectious illness and fever, and modern research has confirmed that it has a sedative effect on the central nervous system. Since it can be a skin irritant, it is best used diluted with a carrier oil. It is good for athlete's foot and skin fungus, against scabies, and as an insect repellent. It helps muscle pains, circulation problems, and, massaged across the abdomen, it helps colitis, indigestion, and gastroenteritis. In India, this oil is reputed to help keep skin clear and healthy and to be effective in treating acne. It raises the spirits and is excellent for depression. It is a good oil to both calm and soothe pittas and to get kaphas moving and into action.

Myrrh

Myrrh is another of the plants that grow throughout Asia and is an essential oil that has been in use for thousands of years. The ancient Egyptians used it as part of their sacred rituals, and it features in the Old and New Testaments, being one of the offerings brought to the infant Jesus by the Magi. Breathing in the aroma of this oil has a drying effect on lung ailments that are producing a lot of mucus and phlegm. So it helps bronchitis, coughs and cold infections, and also sore throats. Its most famous use, even today, is in healing mouth and gum problems—it is great for ulcers, gingivitis, pyorrhea, and other conditions of inflammation. A few drops of myrrh in water make a very effective gargle. Added to massage oil, it will help all kinds of skin problems,

105

from boils and ulcers to bedsores. Massaged across the abdomen, it eases gastritis, diarrhea, and dyspepsia. It is a stimulating oil and therefore good for kapha types.

Orange

Another ancient remedy, the orange tree had its origin in China and has therefore been used for over three thousand years in traditional Chinese medicine. There are two kinds of orange, the sweet and the bitter. Although there is a bitter orange essential oil, it is the sweet orange that is most widely used. The sweet orange tree actually yields three different essential oils—orange from the peel, neroli from the white flowers, and petit grain from the leaves. As befits such a rich array, there are many uses for these oils.

- Sweet orange essential oil added a few drops at a time to water and used for washing the face will brighten dull and listless skin. Added to massage oil, it can be used to reduce obesity and water retention and to help painful joints. Massaged specifically over the abdomen and lower back, it eases constipation and calms dyspepsia and gastric spasms.
- Over the chest and upper back, it eases bronchitis. It raises the body temperature slightly, so using it as an allover massage oil will help drive out chills and fever, as well as encouraging the sweating out of toxins. Breathing in the aroma will calm nausea, especially morning sickness. It has a powerful spirit-lifting capacity and helps those who feel depressed or underenergized. It is at the same time calming and

emotionally warming, and therefore it is good for both vata and pitta types. The special uses of neroli are to calm and relax people and to help brides and grooms to relax and enjoy their sexual beginnings together. Used in massage over the abdomen, it calms disturbed intestines and may help ease the symptoms of diarrhea. Neroli is also a potent skin helper, regenerating skin cells and bringing new life to aging and dry skin. It improves its elasticity and creates a more youthful appearance. Petit grain is used in massage oil to soothe a hyperactive system. It sedates the nervous system, slows the heartbeat, and deepens breathing.

107

Peppermint

This is another essential oil with a very long history, mint plants having been found in the tombs of the pharaohs. Mint also features in Greek mythology, Mentha having been a nymph who was changed into a plant by the god Pluto. The essential oil has an overwhelming aroma and should be used with care and in very small quantities. It should not be used in a whole-body massage but can be applied locally for special purposes, such as pain relief. Nursing mothers should not use it as it may cause their milk to dry up. It must *not* be used by people using homeopathic remedies, since it will antidote the remedy.

Breathe in the oil for colds, flu, and fevers. It clears the lungs and drives up a fever so as to burn it out quickly. Put a few drops in hot water in a bowl, stick your head over this under a towel, and breathe deeply—it helps clear your lungs, stop catarrh, and is great for people with asthma. It is most helpful in dealing with digestive problems. Breathing in the aroma will ease stomach cramps and intestinal spasms. It will almost instantly put a stop to feelings of nausea of whatever origin—morning sickness, travel sickness, or hangover. A drop or two rubbed on the temples will ease a headache rapidly, and a few drops in warm water will help your aching feet as you soak them. A drop on an aching tooth will quiet it down. Used locally in massage oil on the skin, this will remove toxic congestion and allow better circulation. It will fight ringworm, scabies, and localized itching. Ants hate peppermint, so keep them out with a few drops at their usual entrance to your house. Emotionally, mint cools out anger and resentment, lifts depression, and creates energy. Good for pitta types.

108

Pine

From the pine forests of the Himalayas comes this essential oil, which is another of those known to the ancients. The Egyptians, ancient Greeks, and Arabs were all familiar with this powerful healer. It is especially helpful for pulmonary infections—tuberculosis, pneumonia, and bronchitis. Inhaled, it helps with catarrh, asthma, and stuffed-up sinuses.

It is regarded as helpful for skin problems and as an insect repellent. It works against scabies and lice and heals cuts and sores. Added to massage oil, it will help circulation in arthritic joints, ease pain and achiness, and improve poor circulation. Added to bath water, it helps to ease cystitis and urinary infections and is regarded as a kidney cleanser. It is also traditionally thought to be useful in prostrate and gall-bladder problems. Ayurveda finds pine essential oil very useful in clearing conditions due to congested skin, such as psoriasis and eczema. Inhaled, it is stimulating and helps people overcome fatigue and weakness. Since it has the ability to help people feel grounded, it is good for vata folks.

Rosemary

Native to Asia, rosemary has been traditionally used in temple rituals and was burned to drive away the plague and keep out evil spirits. It has many medicinal uses—it can be used for respiratory complaints; circulatory problems; and muscle and joint aches, pains, and sprains. The essential oil can be added to shampoo or used by itself and rubbed into the head. It stimulates hair growth and scalp health and kills lice. In a massage oil, it will ease stiffness and soreness caused by overstrenuous exertions or by rheumatism and arthritis. Rubbed on the chest, it helps asthma and bronchitis. On the abdomen, it eases dyspepsia, liver disorders, and digestive problems. Inhaled, it supports the immune system and fights colds, flu, and infections. In general, it is regarded as a heart stimulant that can normalize low blood pressure. It is a liver decongestant that, in Ayurveda, is used to treat hepatitis and cirrhosis. This is good for kaphas.

Sage

Sage is a Mediterranean native that now grows worldwide and has long been incorporated into the great traditional medicine systems. The Chinese considered it a cure for infertility, and the Romans had great confidence in its powers to heal wounds. NOTE: this is a powerful oil and it can be toxic. *Never* take it internally and avoid its use throughout pregnancy and breast-feeding. It is much wiser to use clary sage, which is largely without such toxicity and has many healing qualities. Inhaled, clary sage oil can lift up the spirits and energize depression. It helps grief and restores memory function. In massage oil rubbed across the abdomen and on the small of the back, it will help uterine problems and painful cramps in the lower back. It will ease digestive cramps and dyspepsia. Add it to shampoo to encourage hair growth and to clear up dandruff and inflammations of the hair follicles. A few drops in very hot water, inhaled beneath a towel, will help asthma and sore throats. This is excellent for kapha types.

Sandalwood

Sandalwood is a tree native to India that has an ancient history in ritual, sacred, and healing traditions. It has been used for about four thousand years. The ancient Egyptians—who were said to have treated gonorrhea with sandalwood oil—and all the great civilizations that lay along the Silk Road knew of it. Sandalwood oil is excellent for skin problems from eczema to aging and drying skin. Add it to rich carrier oils and use it on the face each night and morning. It has the advantage of being completely nonirritating and nonsensitizing. Inhaled, the oil soothes and eases the heart and mind. It helps to bring peace and acceptance and helps to cut the ties of the past. Added to massage oil and rubbed over the kidney region, it has a purifying and anti-inflammatory action. Over the abdomen, it is traditionally said to relieve frigidity and enhance sexual response. A few drops in hot water, inhaled beneath a towel, helps chest infections, sore throats, and dry coughs. It is a good oil for vata and pitta types.

Thyme

Thyme is a powerful healing agent and is best used as an inhalant since it may cause dermal irritation and be toxic for many. This is another oil to raise the spirits and strengthen the nervous system. It helps the lungs when dealing with coughs, colds, bronchitis, laryngitis, asthma, and sore throats. It helps the body fight disease and supports the immune system. Breathing it in may act as a diuretic and help the removal of uric acid, which will ease rheumatism and arthritis. Adding a few drops to shampoo stimulates hair growth and clears up dandruff. Good for kapha types.

Vetiver

Native to India and other parts of Asia, vetiver is an aromatic grass that produces an oil called the "oil of tranquillity" in India. This is due to its calming action. It is regarded as a great helper for the nervous system and cleanses the aura. It fortifies the red blood system and carries oxygen throughout the body. It restores the body back to health. Added to massage oil, it fights stress and depression, and it can also be added to bath water for the same effects. As a massage, it is a good restorative for those suffering from arthritis aches and pains. It is excellent for pitta types.

8

Help for Catastrophic Conditions

There are a number of conditions that Ayurveda may help that are not easily helped in the standard Western medical protocol. Since most of these health conditions really do require an expert's knowledge and intervention, this chapter should be regarded only as an outline of some possibilities for different approaches. Its intent is to show that there may be other useful approaches to some difficult health issues, and that some valuable progress has been made in Ayurveda. Before getting down to individual health issues, it must be reiterated that Ayurveda is not just a study of symptoms. It is a way of looking at the potential balance of a whole human being. Therefore, any approach to any medical problem must include the individual person being realistic about type, balance, and personal needs. No major medical problem can be dealt with without the individual taking full responsibility for revising lifestyle habits when needed. If you have a major health issue, you need to look at your diet and what it should be, your lifestyle and where it needs adjustment to achieve balance. You also need to look at where you plan to put meditation and your spiritual life into this picture, since a good meditation practice is one of the foundations of making a life of harmony. You can, and many people do, meditate for a sense of inner calm and balance without any spiritual intention, if that is your wish.

There are classically considered to be three major causes of serious illness. The first cause is misuse of the mind and body. This category includes all thoughts and actions that breach the natural order of human life: suppression of natural urges like defecation, coughing, sneezing, and so on; sexual excess; and living without regard for the natural balance and respect that you owe life and yourself. Thus, alcohol and drug use are part of this, along with unhealthy emotional choices, and generally behaving badly and keeping bad company. All of this afflicts your well-being. The second cause is any abuse of the five senses, either by neglect or through excess. The third cause is doing things out of season—at the wrong time of the year, the wrong time in your life cycle, or against the natural rhythm of nature itself. There may also be physical symptoms, although these might be occurring at a subtle level. Significant drops in energy, for example, are a sign. A feeling of nausea in the morning on a regular basis means something. Most people know when something is wrong, even if they choose to do nothing or not to get help from their doctor since the illness is still at a subtle level and not immediately discernible by the present medical technology.

When you're feeling ill in this way, you could be aided by an Ayurvedic physician who would have various ways to check these subtle levels. For example, taking the pulse in Ayurveda reveals a lot about the basic balance of a person. The Ayurvedic physician reads three pulse points on the radial artery, all located next to each other. These three represent the three doshas, and an expert pulse reader can diagnose a great deal from this. This is similar to the Chinese method of pulse reading, except that in traditional Chinese medicine your pulse is read six times, each read relating to a major organ of the body.

In reading the Ayurvedic pulse, the right arm is used for men and the left arm for women, and the pulses are located in a row beneath the thumb and along the radial artery. Press down with your first three fingers and you will find three pulses of different strengths.

115

The index finger finds the vata pulse, the middle finger the pitta pulse, and the ring finger the kapha pulse. A skilled diagnostician can read much into the body's condition from the strength, style, and pattern of these pulses, but anyone can find where they are with a little practice.

These pulses are one of the most important ways in which an Ayurvedic practitioner can help you before you become seriously ill. However, here in the West, most people are somewhat unobservant of their health and balance needs and tend to only pay attention when conditions really demand it. All too often this means only noticing when serious illness is present. Because Ayurveda has developed very differently from Western medicine and because it has a history of dealing with certain conditions, it can offer hope when Western medicine sometimes cannot. Remember, however, that no herbal remedy will be truly effective unless you support its action by taking your life in hand and reestablishing balance. Diet, meditation, yoga, and right living are all part of this picture. No health condition, and especially no serious health condition, can improve without that support and change.

ALZHEIMER'S DISEASE

While not claiming to treat Alzheimer's disease, Ayurvedic medicine certainly has several valuable offerings for those afflicted with Alzheimer's disease, or its beginnings.

One is gotu kola, an herb respected for its ability to revitalize and strengthen nervous function while improving memory. It has long been regarded as a rejuvenator, and it is possible that its anti-inflammatory capacity is also part of this. Western studies have confirmed the usefulness of gotu kola in helping those with memory problems. According to Ayurvedic tradition, the use of gotu kola is associated with the crown chakra and the functioning of the pineal gland. The pineal gland is associated with the coming of wisdom in old age.

Withania, known as *ashwagandha* in Hindi, is also famed for its rejuvenating qualities. It restores the exhausted and renews vitality and helps offset nervous exhaustion—all of which are significant factors in the life of anyone who may be developing Alzheimer's disease. Research in India shows that it raises hemoglobin levels, reduces the graying of hair, and helps recovery from chronic illness. It is calming and encourages rest and relaxation, while at the same time enhancing energy and capacity to cope with life. It could be a very powerful helper.

The traditional herb coleus is also able to improve blood flow to the brain and is widely employed as a heart medicine, a use that has been confirmed by modern research. Improved blood flow to the brain could be instrumental in helping to improve and maintain function. Another important helper for brain function is calamus, known as *bacc* in Hindi. It is another of the rejuvenators, considered to revitalize the brain and nervous system. The rhizome of the plant is dried and ground into powder, and it is this powder that is taken as a tonic.

Yet another weapon against undue aging from the Ayurvedic store is the Indian gooseberry, or *Emblica officinalis*. This was first featured in a seventh-century Ayurvedic text that told how a great sage rejuvenated himself by eating this fruit. To this day, it is given to the old to offset the effects of aging.

CANCER

One of the big questions people always have of any traditional healing system is: Can it cure cancer? Obviously, if the answer was a simple yes, probably the whole world would already have heard this, so that is not the easy answer in Ayurveda. However, the Ayurvedic tradition has an extremely detailed written record of its long dealings with cancer and these are interesting to note. For those wishing to avoid cancer, either because of a particular fear or a family tendency, Ayurvedic observations have a lot to teach us. Just as in the English language, Sanskrit uses special terms to refer to tumor growths, usually to do with their site and their appearance, and Ayurvedic doctors were writing in extreme detail about these issues in the seventh century B.C. Their descriptions run very close to those now employed by Western medicine, and there was clearly a sophisticated understanding of the nature of cancer. Ayurveda assumes that cancer comes about as a result of all three of the Tridosha being in imbalance. These energies—vata, pitta, and kapha—are also the control systems of the body and normally they work in coordination. Only when they become very much out of coordination can cancer develop. It is therefore always a whole body disease, even though it appears in one particular site at its first manifestation. We can say that all cancers are considered systemic in Ayurvedic medicine, no matter where in the actual system they appear. Their appearance is a sign that all the three systems are in disarray. This always signals that a total change of life is needed if the person is to recover, and all choices of treatment should support the function of the immune system as fully as possible. To the keen self-observer, these signs of disarray would have been apparent for a considerable length of time. A benign growth is regarded as an indication of disarray in one or two systems, but a malignant growth is a sign that all three are involved.

The text that first described these cancers was written in the fifth century B.C. It is a very detailed approach to understanding what cancer is, and many of its observations still stand today. The cells from which cancers grow are described in Sanskrit as *napunsaka,* which means that they have no natural function in the body. The text goes on to describe the nature, site, and appearance of the different kinds of growths and their significance.

In the seventh century B.C., it was believed that surgery was the only real answer to a cancerous growth because it involved serious disruption in all three energy systems. Herbal medicines were considered to be helpful only in the very beginning stages since all such medicines were used in order to bring about balance in the body. However, in the case of cancer, the balance had already moved so far out of its healthy stage that herbal medicines did not seem strong enough to restore it. They took too long and were too mild in comparison with the out-of-control nature of cancerous growth.

Over the next thousand years, however, Ayurvedic practitioners began working with alchemical processes that involved using minerals, often originally poisonous, but in minute quantities that were rendered harmless by special processing. These became effective in treating some cancers. It is clear that this process has a lot in common with the Western medicinal system of homeopathy in which minute quantities of poisons may be used to deal with symptoms that would arise from actual poisoning, the theory being that "like cures like." Among the minerals used for treatment of cancers were mercury, gold, silver, copper, arsenic, cyanide, and strychnine. Since cancer is considered serious, anyone dealing with it should see a practitioner in order to get a full insight into the condition and what will be needed. For those who wish to avoid its occurrence, being faithful to the body needs of your type is a very important first step in maintaining a cancer-free lifestyle. Cancer is a manifestation of extreme disharmony and this does not happen overnight.

DIABETES

Ayurveda has a long history of treating diabetes with herbal remedies that bring down blood sugar levels. One such remedy is cerasee, or *Momordica charantia,* a climbing plant found throughout Asia containing certain constituents that include an insulin-like peptide that lowers blood sugar levels in both blood and urine. The unripe fruit of the tree is notably useful in treating late-onset diabetes, and Chinese research in the 1980s confirmed its capacity to lower blood sugar levels.

Another great helper in diabetes is Holy Basil, known as *tulsi* in Hindi, which means "matchless." It helps to stabilize blood sugar levels and research studies confirm that it can be very helpful for some people. It can simply be eaten. Jambul, or *Syzygium cumini*, is often prescribed in powder form in India to counter the effects of diabetes. The powder is made from the fruit of the tree, and it has the ability to lower blood sugar levels. The early stages of Type 2 diabetes respond well to jambul, provided it is combined with strict attention to diet. It also helps to treat the frequent urination that may accompany diabetes. Garlic is also effective in lowering blood sugar levels and is therefore also helpful in late-onset diabetes. The juice of the Indian gooseberry is given to diabetics to strengthen the function of the pancreas.

HEART DISEASE

Any affliction of the heart, apart from those a person may be born with, is regarded as resulting from serious disturbance in the emotional life. This is the true seed of all heart disease. Therefore, it would be very important for a heart patient to consider the ways in which imbalance has been a way of life and just how a proper sense of balance can be restored. Right living, right emotional attitudes, yoga, and meditation are a very important part of any health regime for heart patients. There are several great helpers for the heart in Ayurvedic medicine, some of which seem to bring about great improvement in functioning and which, even more excitingly, have been confirmed by the kind of research westerners feel confident about. One is arjuna, used as a heart tonic for thousands of years. Its greatest value seems to be in cases of angina and where blood supply to the heart is poor. Research shows that arjuna reduces blood cholesterol levels and also helps to maintain a regular heartbeat. It actually improves circulation to the heart and is a heart healer. It is not merely something to keep symptoms in check, as is so often the case in Western medicine. It brings about healthy change in functioning. It is the bark of the arjuna tree that is used to make herbal teas, tinctures, and pills. This is one of the many traditional Ayurvedic herbs that modern research has confirmed in its value. It treats heart failure and the edema that can result from congestive heart failure. It improves heart rate and blood pressure and also reduces heart cholesterol levels. It prevents the development of further heart problems.

121

Coleus is another great heart helper. It lowers blood pressure and is regarded as an important heart and circulatory tonic. It is used to treat congestive heart failure and poor blood flow by dilating the blood vessels. Research in India and Germany in the 1970s resulted in isolating one active constituent, called forskolin, which proved to be powerfully able to reduce high blood pressure. Garlic, that great and humble helper, plays a serious part in improving and maintaining heart health. It lowers blood pressure and keeps a person healthy by counteracting infection and inflammation and fighting off illness. Clinical trials in the 1980s have confirmed that garlic does indeed lower blood pressure and also reduces blood lipid levels. It helps keep circulation healthy and prevents strokes by keeping the blood thin. For heart health, garlic is your good friend.

For general improvement of circulation, use fresh ginger, which helps to carry blood to the capillaries. You can just grate a little gingerroot onto your food each day, and you can also make a ginger tea. Take one inch of fresh gingerroot, chop it up, put it into two cups of water, simmer gently until reduced to one cup, then sip the resulting ginger tea. Adding grated ginger to your bath will also improve circulation all over.

HEPATITIS

Western medicine offers very little help to those with hepatitis, and this is becoming a major issue with the spread of untreatable hepatitis C, regarded as a chronic liver condition that becomes fatal. In fact, some of the treatments are pretty fatal, too. Chemotherapy has been one of the recent choices, a treatment which of course wipes out the immune system and loads even more toxins into an already compromised liver. Traditional Ayurvedic treatment for hepatitis includes the use of healing herbs and the taking of fresh-squeezed lemon juice in a glass of hot water each morning. I underwent these treatments when I had hepatitis while living in Kathmandu, and my hepatitis cleared up really fast—within one week—and I have never had any liver complications from that day to this.

The most well-known herb used for treatment of liver problems in Ayurveda is chiretta, known as *chirayata* in Hindi, and a member of the Gentianaceae family. Native to India and Nepal, it is extremely bitter—a sure sign that it is good for the liver—and contains amarogentin, as well as other active constituents. Amarogentin has been the subject of research in India, and it has demonstrated its special powers to protect the liver. Chiretta increases blood flow to the liver, reduces fever, and is a powerful tonic remedy.

Another powerful liver herb is *Picrorrhiza kurroa*, from the Scrophulariaceae family, which is a mountain herb native to India, Nepal, and Tibet. Its root is routinely used to treat a wide range of liver problems, including jaundice, hepatitis, cirrhosis, and all conditions where a severely compromised immune system is part of the picture. Recent research in India has confirmed these uses and has further suggested that it could be very useful in autoimmune diseases and conditions where a lowered immune system is the major issue. Since this is a particularly powerful herb, it should be taken under professional supervision only.

123

A third great helper is turmeric, known in Hindi as *haldi*. Most people in the West know it only as a spice, but it has long been known in India as a treatment for digestive and liver problems. In the last two decades, laboratory research in India has confirmed these traditional uses in a convincing series of studies. It is also a powerful anti-inflammatory, shown in studies to be more powerful than the extremely damaging drug hydrocortisone. It has a protective action on the stomach and liver. Just grate the dried root and take one teaspoon of the resulting powder in water three times a day.

Another extremely valuable helper for liver problems is licorice. One of its key constituents, glycyrrhizine, has been demonstrated in laboratory research to be an effective treatment for chronic hepatitis and liver cirrhosis. It can be taken as dried powder, a whole plant tincture, or as dried root that can be chewed. If using the tincture, you might want to drop it into very hot water and let that stand overnight so that all the alcohol is evaporated.

KIDNEY STONES

Ayurvedic medicine offers a great helper and healer for kidney stones—the varuna tree. It is becoming very exciting for Western medicine, too, since research is backing up how very useful it is. The bark of the tree has active constituents that have been demonstrated to help the bladder, prevent the formation of stones, and reduce the rate at which possible stone-forming elements are deposited in the kidneys. Thus, it seems to provide a control of the process. Varuna is being given to patients in the West now to both prevent and treat kidney stones. It is also prescribed for those who already have small stones, since it improves functioning of the bladder and enables it to pass stones with much less pain and trauma.

Remember that all serious conditions require a complete change of life, from revising the way you eat to changing your job if it does not support your real health. Additionally, Ayurveda regards it as essential that you take up yoga and meditation as part of bringing back that much-needed harmony into your life. There is no such thing as profound good health without paying attention to your spiritual and emotional needs for balance and harmony. Your only protection is to have harmony, order, and balance in all aspects of your energy systems—body, mind, spirit, and consciousness. In fact, ill health is one of the most desperate ways that your body calls your attention to the fact that something is wrong with your life. So, if this is you, wake up—wake up and live.

The Panchakarma
Healing Regime

Much of Ayurveda is concentrated on finding and maintaining balance in life, achieved through the fairly gentle regimes of diet, exercise, meditation, and living within the comfort zones of one's type. If there are major problems to be dealt with, however, the radical cleansing routines of the Panchakarma have to be applied. Literally, Panchakarma means "five actions," and it refers to the cleansing out of toxins from the body by stimulating the natural ways in which the body rejects toxins. It is done when abnormal accumulations of energy are causing disease. In the culture of India, this is not regarded as especially rigorous, since complex cleansing rituals—inside and out—are already part of the Hindu culture and practice. However, most westerners are likely to look at this somewhat askance. There is no doubt that this kind of profound cleaning out of toxins is a powerful way to deal with the major illnesses such as cancer and kidney and liver disease that develop as a result of such toxins.

The five techniques of Panchakarma are:

1. Therapeutic vomiting or *vamana*.
2. Purgation or *virechana*.
3. Enemas or *basti*.
4. Nasal application of herbs or *nasya*.
5. Bloodletting or *raktamokshana*.

Traditionally, people are supposed to do this three times a year for best results at the beginning of certain seasons—spring, fall, and winter. Even in India, however, this practice has become much less common. It mainly takes place now in Ayurvedic retreat centers which, by Indian economic standards, are costly and therefore largely the provenance of the rich. Ordinary people on the whole no longer include these ritual cleansings in their life. They are unlikely to appeal to most westerners either, but if they were your only resource to deal with serious illness, then you would be likely to consider undertaking such a demanding regime.

VAMANA

Vomiting therapy removes excess kapha energy from the stomach and the lungs. This energy in excess creates mucus and phlegm and allows illnesses like asthma and bronchitis to develop. To bring about therapeutic vomiting, the patient drinks up to six cups of an herbal mixture, which typically includes some or all of the following—lobelia, *Nux vomica*, licorice, or pennyroyal. Then the patient is supposed to induce vomiting by rubbing the back of the tongue. This is usually done once a day for several days, first thing in the morning on an empty stomach, but it can also be done just once for good therapeutic effect. It is considered to be very effective in treating fevers of recent origin, bronchial asthma, sinusitis, skin diseases, upper respiratory tract diseases, goiter, obesity, abscesses, epilepsy, tumors, anemia, and diabetes. It should not be done by anyone who is elderly, pregnant, menstruating, or suffering from certain illnesses such as heart problems, nervous disorders, tuberculosis, eye conditions, vertigo, retention of urine, or headaches. After this treatment, the patient feels less pain in the body, more clarity of mind, and a general sense of lightness.

127

VIRECHANA

Purgation therapy begins by the patient taking ghee (clarified butter) for several days in a row first thing in the morning. This is called oleation therapy or *sneehana*. It dampens the appetite and prepares the body for purgative therapy, basically by softening the stool. Then the patient swallows a laxative herbal drink that might include any or all of the following: castor oil, senna leaf tea, aloe vera juice or gel, *Cascara segrada*, rhubarb, dandelion, or psyllium seed infusion. This encourages the whole intestinal tract to empty itself, which lowers pitta energy and reduces the digestive fires further. Different recipes for the purgation therapy are used, according to the individual patient, the season of the year, and of course the conditions of health presented by the patient. This would be suitable for all patients *except* those suffering from any of the following: fever, abdominal pain, diarrhea, ulcerative colitis or irritable bowel syndrome, alcoholism, tuberculosis, colds, obesity with constipation, or prolapse of the rectum. It is especially useful for those who have any of the following conditions: urinary disorders, enlargement of the spleen, toxemia, elephantiasis, chronic ulcers, burns, edema, abscesses, gynecological disorders, epilepsy, headaches, and insanity. For people who have long-term constipation, bile problems, or an excess of mucus, hot pungent herbs are used. For others, herbs that are cooling and bring about sweating are used.

The ancient text *Caraka Samhita* devotes six chapters to the herbs used in purgation therapy, and a different set is used for each person. There are special recipes for purgation against poisoning, another for hemorrhoids, and even a purgative especially for aristocratic people. Others are seasonal recipes—for the rainy season, for the end of the rainy season, for winter, for summer. Others are for body types—obese people, dehydrated people, and there is even a special laxative wine. Purgative herbs remove excess pitta from the stomach and the entire body. Purgation therapy eradicates diseases and restores normal strength and complexion. It extends the length of your life, clears the brain, and strengthens the senses and the locomotor system. Digestion improves.

BASTI

Medicated enemas have long been not only an elimination practice in Ayurveda but often an actual form of treatment for many kinds of diseases or troubling symptoms. Among these can be any of the following: constipation, arthritis, anxiety, headaches, viral infections, and lower back pain. They can also help a wide range of other conditions, such as enlargement of the spleen, elephantiasis, eye diseases, chronic ulcers, burns, edema, abscesses, gout, gynecological disorders, and jaundice. There are over one hundred different formulas for medical enemas, and they may include mixes of oils such as sesame, castor, or herbalized oil. They may be concoctions of water or milk including herbs like calamus, triphala, ginger, licorice, or gotu kola. They may even be made from broths of meat and bone marrow.

Enemas in Ayurvedic medicine are not necessarily administered via the rectum. In fact, there are four possible sites for enemas. The first is via the rectum. The second is via the vagina or penis, having an action on the urinary bladder. The third is through the vagina to the uterus, and the fourth is at the site of ulcers, bringing about cleansing and healing. People with the following conditions would not be advised to take enema therapy: piles, cholera, intestinal obstruction, vomiting, severe dyspepsia, skin diseases, diabetes, and pregnancy.

NASYA

Nasal administration of medicinal herbs removes excess kapha energy from the head and neck regions. The nose passes signals directly to the limbic system brain, the part of the brain that most powerfully controls our emotions and central nervous system. Herbs absorbed via the nose have a very rapid effect on the emotional system, while the active-ingredient molecules enter the lungs and are absorbed directly into the bloodstream. Therefore, using the nasal administration of herbs is a rapid way to jump-start the body into balance and healing. It is considered to be a very effective way to treat conditions that have a strong emotional component, and, of course, it also purifies the nose, sinus cavities, throat, and head of toxins and infections.

In nasya, the herbs are used in powder, paste, or oil form, and the fresh juice of many of the plants can also be used directly. First, the patient has oil massaged on his or her face, head, neck, and shoulders for ten minutes or so. Then the area is washed with hot water for about five minutes, and the patient then lies down and his head is supported so that his nose is up and the top of his head down. This makes it easy to administer the herbs nasally. Four to eight drops of fresh plant juice can be placed in each nostril or powder can be administered. This is done by filling one end of an open-ended tube with tightly packed medicinal powder, sticking that end in the nostril, and having the physician blow hard so that the powder enters the nostril. It is also possible to make a boiling pot of the medical decoction so that the patient breathes in the steam.

Many herbs and oils are used in nasya. Among the powders are calamus root, gotu kola, ginger, and chilis. Ghee, aloe vera juice, sesame oil, onion juice, basil juice, and milk are often used. This treatment can be used in cases of colds, headaches, facial paralysis, nervous disorders, neuralgia, and many other cranial and cervical conditions, as well as for strengthening the veins, arteries, nerves, joints, ligaments, and tendons of the neck and head. It usually produces a cheerful, upbeat mood, a good voice, stronger sensory organs, and hair that resists turning gray.

It promotes memory, power, and intelligence, and immunizes the body against viral and bacterial infections. The head feels clear. The patient sleeps well.

RAKTAMOKSHANA

Bloodletting lets out impure blood in small quantities in order to release toxins and expel excess pitta energy from the lymph and blood. Traditionally, this was done either by using a cutting instrument or by using leeches. Bloodletting stimulates the immune system and helps to overcome imbalances caused mainly by incorrect lifestyles. These include sleeping after meals, sleeping in the daytime, giving way to excessive anger, excessive exposure to sunlight, suppression of natural urges like defecation, and excessive exercise. Another cause is eating wrongly—too much unwholesome or pungent food; too many acid foods; too much meat, vinegar, or sour foods; rotten food; and foods improper for your energy type. According to the ancient texts, there are over sixty diseases of the blood that show up with a variety of symptoms, such as acid indigestion, excessive sleep, myalgia, anorexia, vertigo, skin conditions, thirst, bad breath, conjunctivitis, and pyorrhea.

The best time for bloodletting, say the medical texts, is a pleasant and auspicious day that is neither too hot nor too cold nor too cloudy. Bloodletting should not be done in the rainy season or when the sky is cloudy. These days, bloodletting is uncommon and never done in this country. Purification is usually done by the use of herbal therapies now.

There are other preparations that may precede the Panchakarma and they include:

- *Sneehana* karma or oleation therapy, which means using oil massage to make the skin smooth, moist, and relaxed. Using sesame oil, the patient is massaged for half an hour or so. Using massage oil every day is good for health, longevity, the complexion, and the eyes, and it helps a person sleep well, too. Different herbs are added to the oil, individualized for each person. Another version of this therapy has the patient lie down in a bed of oil for up to half an hour. This is a rejuvenation therapy and is also great for mental disorders.

  It is also not unlike the healing rituals of the ancient Greeks at the sacred healing temple of the god Aesculapius, the god of healing. In these, the sick were made to lie on a stone bed filled with medicinal oils all night in the sacred atmosphere of the temple. The god Aesculapius visited them in their dreams and gave guidance on how they could find their health again. In the morning, the temple healer-priests would help them to interpret their dreams.
- *Swedana:* Sweating therapy consists of using herbalized steam to open up the pores and let impurities out.
- *Shirodhara:* This treatment consists of slowly dripping warm sesame oil infused with healing herbs onto the Third Eye area between the eyebrows. This induces a light trance and allows a person to become deeply and completely relaxed and peaceful. When done by an Ayurvedic practitioner, other decoctions may be

used—milk with herbal remedies infused in it, buttermilk, or sugarcane juice. This is one way in which people with serious mental disorders are helped.

ABHYANGA

Self-massage every day before your bath or shower is a great gift to yourself and to your present and future health. Doing this helps you live longer, builds strength, helps your complexion, relieves fatigue, tones up the eyesight, and helps you sleep well.

It is best to use refined sesame oil (not the Chinese cooking kind, which has been processed), available from your local health food or organic store. This is not only an enriching treatment for your skin, but it activates the vital energy points all over your body, the *marma* points. The marma points are a network of 107 vital energy points through which easy flow of prana must be maintained in order to maintain balance and health. According to the ancient text *Sushruta Samhita*, marma points are where two or more important anatomical parts meet—blood vessels, bones, nerves, ligaments, muscles, or joints. These create a concentrated energy site. If the flow of prana, or energy, is obstructed in one or more marma points, disease will result. Massage helps to maintain flow, which in turn keeps the whole being in balance.

There are oils particularly suitable for each type:

- For vatas—sesame, olive, almond, wheat germ, and castor.

133

- For pittas—coconut, sandalwood, pumpkin seed, almond, and sunflower.
- For kaphas—sesame, safflower, corn.

Sesame oil makes a wonderful everyday massage oil for all types, since each major type also contains vata energy, and it is this which most responds to the nurturing of daily massage. Before using your oil, heat it up gently in a bowl of very hot water. Make sure your bathroom floor is protected since it is almost impossible not to drop some of the oil. Then lie down and relax for a few minutes while the oil continues to warm up to at least body temperature. Take several long deep breaths and set all your worries and concerns aside. This is to be your time for yourself, a period of nurturing that will enrich your whole day. Undress and begin your massage at the head and then work your way down to your feet. Start by pouring a tablespoon of oil on your head and rub it in using the palm of your hand, not the fingers. Make little circles of movement all over your scalp, then move to your face and ears using lighter movements. Don't forget the back of your ears and your temples. Using fingers and palms together, work on your neck and shoulders. Work more energetically on arms, using circular motions at your shoulders and elbows. For the long bones of the body, work up and down in long strokes. With gentle circular movements, work on the abdomen, chest, and stomach in clockwise direction. Reach behind you and use long up-and-down strokes on as much of your back as you can reach. Use more vigor on your legs, with circular movements at the knees and ankles, and long up-and-down strokes between. Finally, vigorously work on your feet, using the palms of your hands on the foot itself and your fingers on your toes. When you bathe, do not scrub too vigorously but try to keep a light layer of the sesame oil on your skin. It will protect you against aging and wear and tear, and it also protects your spiritual and emotional well-being. It is very settling for all that vata nervous energy.

Ayurvedic tradition regards the skin as one of the seats of vata energy, with a direct energy connection to the main seat of vata in the large intestine. Daily massage stimulates circulation and soothes the nerves while also toning the actions of the major organs of the body. To get the full effects and benefits of self-massage, you must do it mindfully, concentrating as you do it.

135

DINACHARYA
(Daily Health Care Habits)

You are probably not surprised by now to learn that Ayurvedic wisdom has clear ideas on how best to live your life, and a balancing, steady routine is the healthiest way to do this. Moreover, this routine should be closely allied with the natural rhythms of the world itself, so that your life is supported and nurtured by the power of nature itself. We should, say the sages, rise at an early and regular hour and conduct our day in harmony with the universe so that we strengthen our energy and keep ourselves pure, healthy, and happy. Constant change and stimulation is not the key to harmony or happiness. According to the ancient texts, we should rise between 5 A.M. and 6 A.M., just before sunrise. Then we should empty our bladder and bowels. To help things along, if this is earlier than your usual pattern of elimination, you can drink a glass of warm water. This acts as a stimulant to the muscles of the intestines and gets them ready to do their work. After that, clean teeth and tongue and wash the face. Ayurvedic texts, and Dr. Deepak Chopra, recommend a drop of sesame oil be inhaled into each nostril every morning at this time to protect the body against diseases entering via the eyes, ears, and nose. It is also said to be good for all connective tissues in the upper part of the body. Gargle and then trim and clean nails and, for men, shave. Follow this with the abhyanga, or self-massage, with sesame oil, and then some harmonious form of exercise. If you cannot exercise at this time, then late afternoon before dinner would be an appropriate time to choose. Take your bath or shower, put on clean clothes, and meditate. After this, it is time for breakfast.

Near sunset, meditate again. Have your evening meal, take a short walk, spend your evening time harmoniously and quietly. Go to sleep before 10 P.M. Traditional teachings on maintaining health and harmony also emphasize how useful and helpful to your body it is to fast one day a week. It is not only that fasting cuts down how much you eat—a major factor with all the processed foods in modern life—but that one day a week your agni, or digestive fire, is not engaged in working on food. This means it is free to start work on the toxins that have gathered in your digestive tract. Thus, fasting is also a powerful way of cleansing.

There are many ways to fast, from doing a strict water-only fast (probably not a bad thing for most of us) to doing juice, herbal tea, or fruit fasts. Fasting for one day a week is good for all three dosha types. However, vata and pitta people should never go beyond three days of fasting. Vata is increased by fasting and quickly becomes unbalanced, something that vata people already tend toward. Pitta people quickly become irritable, bad-tempered, and even dizzy with fasting. If you do a water-only fast, be sure to use spring or well water. Good teas for fasting are single herb teas—avoid blends since they bring together too many different energies, which is not useful to your body during fasting. Good choices are ginger, dandelion, cardamom, and raspberry. Good choices for juices are the vegetable juices. Drink plenty, more than you feel you want to, anything up to a gallon a day would not be too much. It would be especially good on your fasting days to also work with the essential oils that calm the doshas. Use them purely as aromatherapy on those days, either through an electrical diffuser or using the time-honored candle and aroma-pot method. The pots are small pottery, ceramic, or metallic containers under which you can put a tea-light sized candle, add water to the pot, and then four to six drops of essential oil. These work for several hours at a time.

- Vata-calming oils include basil, cedarwood, geranium, juniper, lavender, myrrh, patchouli, and ylang-ylang.
- Pitta-calming oils include jasmine, lavender, lotus, rose, sandalwood, and vetiver.
- Kapha-calming oils include basil, eucalyptus, frankincense, lemon, peppermint, and rosemary.

In the many centuries since the forming of Ayurvedic teachings about health and harmony, we have moved far. The society we live in now would seem to have little in common with that far-off and long-ago society of the Indus Valley. We would probably rather do anything than follow the demands of the Panchakarma. Even in India, it has become less commonly done. If we are unwell, we prefer to do something easy, like take a pill. However, we seem to be reaching a point in our history where that once-easy solution is no longer easy or even safe. Arguably this is partly because what was once the medical profession has been largely hijacked by the drug trade. Never before have doctors been so ignorant of the substances with which they treat their patients. Imagine the state of medicine if doctors only went by the recommendation of the salesmen selling drugs. Well, that is exactly where we are right now. This is why over half of all hospitalizations of people over age sixty-five are connected with their medications, not with their diseases. Also, doctors are actually falling behind in success with treating illnesses that we might describe as energy illnesses. Cancer figures are at an all-time high, with treatments becoming so horrific that they are actually worse than the disease. Enormous numbers of people have allergies, and more people than ever are dying of asthma. The autoimmune conditions are increasing all the time—lupus, irritable bowel syndrome, chemical sensitivities, hepatitis C, fibromyalgia, and chronic fatigue. Not only are they increasing, but Western mainstream medicine has little or even nothing useful to offer.

No doubt we could speculate about a thousand different reasons for the increase in these illnesses—undoubtedly disharmony in the world and disharmony within ourselves are the two greatest causes. Most importantly, though, people want to know what to do. This is where Ayurveda comes up with some hope and some suggestions. It outlines the ways in which we each need to live, eat, and help ourselves and also offers spiritual and emotional guidance, as well as physical fitness. It even offers the Panchakarma for those who are seriously out of balance, and you don't have to go to India to experience this kind of help since there are a number of Ayurvedic treatment and health centers right here in the United States. So, if you feel that you are suffering from what is really an energy illness, something that started after a shock or a trauma of some kind, or something that has come about after a long period of not really living your life the way you might like to, take a good look at what Ayurveda and its treatments might have to offer you.

10

Nurturing the Spirit: Meditation and Yoga

As we have seen, Ayurveda seeks to help the human find balance in every aspect of life, from the physical to the metaphysical, and two of its most precious ways of nurturing the spirit is through meditation and through the practice of yoga. Meditation has become a familiar part of many people's spiritual lives in recent decades, and those who have never practiced it have at least heard about it. It has even returned to become part of Christianity again, and it always was the integral part of several Eastern religions. However, it is not necessary to be a spiritual believer to gain the benefits of meditation. It is true that Ayurvedic sages would have been astonished to come upon human beings who were disengaged in spiritual practice of any kind. The whole essence of Ayurveda was that the human being needed to be as much in balance as possible in order to fully experience the joining of consciousness with the Absolute. It is probably fair to say that a person with no spiritual life certainly lacks many layers of awareness that others have, but it is still true that meditation has something to offer even the atheist and the nonbeliever.

What exactly does meditation do? Basically, it slows down the hectic energy of the human mind—the part that sages call the monkey mind because it is always leaping about and chasing after nothing much, like monkeys do. Another way to think of meditation is to see it as a way of bringing serenity to the rough ocean of our emotions, so that we can begin to see some other truths working in our lives. Most human beings are fully occupied in reacting to events and people. This makes it easy for us to assume that we are what we feel. Meditation teaches us that we are more than the sum of our feelings. That our feelings, in fact, are not a very true guide to who we are. They change, like the waves of the ocean, ebbing and flowing, just as our wants and desires change. In fact, most of the things that occupy the superficial surface of our thoughts have very little to do with who we really are. The problem is the way we live now seldom allows us to come to that realization.

Living as we do, surrounded by movement and sound, and with the demands of our lives that make us go here, do this, meet her, eat that, we scarcely know who we really are or what we really want. The complexity of modern life is very destructive to our real, basic, deep nature. This is one of the main reasons we are looking at such an epidemic of what we might call energy illnesses—lupus, fibromyalgia, allergies, cancers. Meditation can begin to save us from our superficialities. It can bring us home to ourselves. Once we begin to slow down our minds, we have given ourselves the sacred space in which we can begin to learn the nature of our consciousness. We can begin to see ourselves with true discernment. Some of what we see, we may not like at first, but meditating gives us the power to change what we do not like. In its stillness is our strength. Many people also find that they have sacred revelations in that precious stillness, that they can come to a real comprehension of the nature of the sacred and to a communion with the divine. In this stillness, we can come to states of happiness and bliss that we did not realize were possible. We can understand our true nature, that part of us which is deep and unchanging and has wisdom, and it can speak to us more and more. In Buddhism this is called becoming enlightened. This does not mean that people change utterly and forever, always living in some exalted state. Basically, it means returning to live an ordinary life in an extraordinary way because insight has put us in continuing connection with wisdom. It means living in the spirit of continuing love.

143

That is what enlightenment is—awakening to love and moving to live from the heart instead of from the head. But suppose this is not what you want; that what you want is just some way to feel a bit more in charge of yourself, a bit more balanced, and a bit less thrown about by life; less stressed, more happy. You can get that from meditation, too.

You do not have to be in any way religious to meditate. You do not have to become a follower of any Eastern religion. You can meditate even if you are a fundamentalist Christian. There is nothing very outlandish about meditation. It is simply a discipline you can learn to wind down your overactive mind. Suppose you want to reduce your angina pain or lessen your migraine attacks. You can get that from meditation. The practice of meditation can be done at any level you want. In fact, in recent years there have been many studies of the benefits of meditation, and many of those benefits are very material. You can lower your blood pressure through meditation. You can reduce the number of asthma attacks you have. You can have fewer heart attacks. You can reduce your feelings of stress and become better able to get a good night's sleep. You can start the day off better, so you perform better at work. It can be that simple.

There are many ways to meditate, and resources are given in the resources section on how to do so, but here is a very simple way to start. This is actually the way the Buddha taught his disciples to meditate, but anyone can try it because it is so simple. If you can sit comfortably cross-legged on a cushion, do so. Otherwise, sit upright on a straight-backed chair, not leaning against the back. Keep your back as straight as you can but also try to keep the muscles relaxed. Fold one hand upon the other, both palms facing upward and settle them in your lap at the base of your belly. Close your eyes. Begin to breathe deliberately, as slowly as you can. Be aware of the movement of your body as that breath goes in and out. If stray thoughts come—and they will—observe them, let them go, and continue to concentrate on your breath going in and out. Center your attention on the breath below your naval. Keep breathing, keep sitting, keep letting go of stray thoughts, coming back to your breathing, and do this for as long as you can. Fifteen minutes would make a great start—and will probably seem endless. However, once you try this, you will soon notice that you are much calmer, that you feel much more sensible and less easily thrown about in your emotions and your wants and fears. You will probably begin to see other changes in the way you view the world and even in your values, but that will be up to you. Some meditation teachers refer to this feeling as "coming home to your heart," which is a very descriptive way to show its importance.

Meditation has many forms. Every spiritual tradition has its own kind of meditation. Tibetan Mahayana Buddhism teaches people to visualize extremely complex cultural images as a way of mastering this monkey mind of ours, images that have great depth and meaning for Tibetans and students of Tibetan Buddhism. The older, simpler tradition of Theravada or southern Buddhism, which many say is much closer to the practice of Buddha himself, teaches meditation through breathing. Hinduism, the culture out of which the Buddha came, has some very complex meditation practices using breathing practices and mantras, or sacred words used repetitively. Meditation in the Christian tradition usually involves silent prayer or dialogue with God or Christ. The easiest form of meditation to begin with is breathing meditation. Sit quietly, upright and yet relaxed, and breathe in and out. You can think to yourself as you do it, "I am breathing in," as you breathe in, "I am breathing out," as you breathe out. The point of saying these words in your mind is to help you focus on the breathing.

You'll soon find that the hardest thing is trying to keep track of your thoughts at all. You might manage for a moment or two but then you will start to reminisce about something, replay a scene with someone, think about the bird singing outside your window, anything rather than concentrate only on your breathing. All of this is very normal. This is exactly why we

145

need to meditate, because we can hardly ever keep our minds from running around in this way. Yet we do not experience peace of mind until we can do so. That is what peace of mind is. It is not so much living without the drama and workloads and demands made on us, as it is finding time for peace in our minds no matter what the external distractions. The biggest lie most people tell themselves is that they will relax when they have everything done and have no problems. But that is called being dead. That is virtually the only time you will be done with everything and have no more earthly problems. Life is demands and problems. You do not have to wait for all those things to go away before you find peace. You can sit down right now and find it by watching your breath go steadily in and out. We often feel so overwhelmed by life—especially these days when we are so busy with largely unimportant things—that we cannot imagine taking control of our time, our feelings, and our state of mind. However, meditation gives us exactly that opportunity. And we can do it any time we choose.

Traditionally, Ayurvedic wisdom suggests that the best times of the day for meditation are between 5 and 6 A.M. and then again at twilight. And so they are. You will find your meditation going so much better if you can follow these hours. However, any time you can find will be better than none. And you don't have to be somewhere special and private to do this, although a special quiet place is best. You could be sitting on a bus and meditating. You could even be in your doctor's office. You could be anywhere you can sit still and close your eyes with your hands folded naturally on your lap. This automatically changes your life into one where no minute is wasted or lost.

As you focus your breathing, this will gradually bring about great change in your life. It will enable you to relax, to become centered and grounded, and to feel as if you really can take control of your life. That will allow the development of spiritual richness that you might otherwise have never found in your life. The form that these riches take will depend upon how you choose to develop your meditation. There are many paths leading to full spiritual realization and one destination—the heart. The rest will be revealed as you journey.

YOGA

Yoga typifies the way in which Ayurvedic wisdom regards exercise, compared with the usual western way. Yoga is a gently demanding rhythmic series of movements that aim to harmonize the whole body until its perfection becomes a spiritual attainment. There is almost no western form of exercise that can match it. Indeed, the most common forms of western exercise are the exact opposite of harmonizing. Contact sports tend to be violent and often physically damaging in a major way, built upon personal ego. Running and jogging are for the adrenaline-addicted, and are deeply damaging to the structure and health of the physical body. Only walking comes close to the Ayurvedic ideal.

One of Ayurveda's greatest gifts to the West is the practice of yoga, a form of exercise the aim of which is to restore circulation, flow, harmony, and balance to the whole body at all its levels of being. Ideally, you need to attend a class and you can be sure that, wherever you live in the United States, someone is

147

offering a yoga class. It may be a local church, your community college, a gym, or a private individual, but someone is doing it near where you live. If you really cannot get to or find such a class, there are some excellent videos available, and these are listed in the resources section at the end of the book.

In the meantime, think about adding the Salute to the Sun to your morning wake-up session for yourself.

Resources

INSTITUTES OF AYURVEDIC STUDIES

American Institute of Vedic Studies
Director: Dr. David Frawley
P.O. Box 8357
Santa Fe, NM 87504
(505) 983-9385

This institute offers an Ayurvedic correspondence course.

The Ayurvedic Institute & Wellness Center
Director: Dr. Vasant Lad
P.O. Box 23445
Albuquerque, NM 87192-1445
(505) 291-9698

This institute offers a wide range of services, education, and Ayurvedic resources. It has a nine-month study program, which includes an Ayurvedic studies program. The program consists of 700 hours of class-room instruction in its first year.

The "Gurukula" program (2d, 3rd, and 4th academic year) offers 350 hours of study per year. In addition to these, the institute also offers special summer intensive seminars, weekend seminars, as well as a correspondence course by Robert Svoboda, B.A.M.S.

The Panchakarma department offers traditional Ayurvedic procedures for purification and rejuvenation that include oil massage, herbal steam treatment, shirodhara, cleansing diet, herbal therapy, lifestyle education, and other therapies. The institute also maintains an herbal and healing products department offering Ayurvedic and western herbs for sale.

The institute maintains a comprehensive on-line database of Ayurvedic and western herbs and food substances examined through the three-thousand-year-old clinical eyes of Ayurveda.

The institute's Ayurved Press primarily publishes the books and articles of Dr. Lad and Dr. Svoboda, but it also publishes other traditional Ayurvedic and Vedic works.

150

The California College of Ayurveda
Director: Marc Halpern, D.C., C.A.S.
1117A East Main Street
Grass Valley, CA 95945
(530) 274-9100

This is the first state-approved college for the study of Ayurvedic medicine in the country. It offers education and training in the new profession of Clinical Ayurvedic Specialist (C.A.S.).

The California College of Ayurveda is dedicated to giving the student the finest education within the field of Ayurveda. Its two-year program is rigorous, yet designed to accommodate individuals who are juggling busy schedules or who live at a distance.

Combining classroom education with independent study, the program culminates in a supervised six-month internship either in the student's community or at the college's Ayurvedic community health care clinic.

The college is recognized by the Ayurved/Shikshan Mandal, a government-authorized accrediting agency in India, and by the American Institute of Vedic Studies. An additional internship in India is available to course graduates through the International Academy of Ayurveda.

PROFESSIONAL ASSOCIATIONS

International Federation for Ayurveda
13 West 9th Street
New York, NY 10011
(212) 505-8971

American Holistic Medical Association
4101 Lake Boone Trail, Suite 201
Raleigh, NC 27607
(919) 787-5181

AYURVEDIC TREATMENT
CENTERS AND SPAS

151

Canyon Ranch
Tucson, Arizona
1-800-742-9000 for more information

This spa offers a variety of Ayurvedic treatments, plus Ayurvedic herbal rejuvenation.

The Center for Thai Massage
Mill Valley, California
(415) 388-1870 for more information

A day spa based on Indian Ayurvedic medicine, Buddhist spiritual practice, and yoga; offering Thai massage.

The Chopra Center for Well-Being
7630 Fay Avenue
La Jolla, CA 92037
(858) 551-7788; 1-888-424-6772
Fax: (858) 551-7811
E-mail: info@chopra.com

A resort spa with a comprehensive Ayurvedic program. The center has Ayurvedic treatments to enliven the connection between body, mind, emotions, and spirit; reduce stress; increase creativity; restore vitality; and enhance strength.

The Fallbrook Wellness Spa
123 East Alvarado Street
Fallbrook, CA 92028
(760) 723-8264
Fax: (760) 723-7834
E-mail: fallbrook@wellnessspa.com

Consultation determines which herbs, oils, and creams will be appropriate for the predominant doshas for the person at that time. Offers a range of Ayurvedic treatments.

Watercourse Way
165 Channing Avenue
Palo Alto, CA 94301
(650) 462-2000

It is a day spa offering a variety of Ayurvedic rejuvenating treatments.

The Raj Maharishi Ayur-Ved Health Center
Fairfield, Iowa
1-800-742-9000 for more information

This resort spa offers Ayurvedic massage, transcendental meditation, stress management, self-pulse diagnosis, skin care, nutrition, diet counseling, internal cleansing, and more.

National Institute of Ayurvedic Medicine
584 Milltown Road
Brewster, NY 10509
(914) 278-8700

Dr. Gerson's Manhattan office:
13 West 9th Street
New York, NY 1001
(212) 505-897

This resort spa offers four- and eight-day retreats in the residential Panchakarma Retreat Center, and it is also a research facility and center for workshops. It has an herb garden, research library, and teaching kitchen. The NIAM is located in Brewster, New York, sixty miles north of Manhattan, on six and one half acres of land.

The National Institute of Ayurvedic Medicine (NIAM) is recognized as the largest and most authentic resource of information on Ayurveda in the United States. It was established in 1982 by Scott Gerson, M.D., who holds degrees in both Ayurveda and conventional allopathic medicine. Dr. Gerson's medical practice has combined Ayurveda and conventional medicine for more than fifteen years.

Many medicinal plants used in Ayurveda grow in the center's herb garden as well as throughout the property. The NIAM Research Library contains one of the largest collections of Ayurvedic literature in the United States and includes writings and research reports in English, Hindi, Sanskrit, Malayalam, Tamil, and several other dialects.

153

The Ayurvedic Center
4100 Westheimer, Suite 235
Houston, TX 77027
(713) 661-9760
Fax: (713) 663-7307

This is a day spa that offers Ayurvedic consultations to explore causes of physical or emotional discomfort from a holistic perspective in order to arrive at the best path for a return to health and happiness.

AYURVEDIC HERBAL SUPPLIERS

Banyan Trading Company *(Wholesale Practitioner Prices)*
P.O. Box 13002
Albuquerque, NM 87192
(505) 244-1878; 1-800-953-6424
Web site: www.banyantrading.com

Bazaar of India Imports *(Wholesale Practitioner Prices)*
1810 University Avenue
Berkeley, CA 94703
1-800-261-7662
E-mail: info@ayur-veda.com

Ask about Bazaar of India's practitioner services package (includes special practitioner pricing, no minimums, custom labeling to your specs, free delivery, empty dispensing bottles, and much more).

Lotus Light *(Wholesale Prices)*
P.O. Box 325
Twin Lakes, WI 53181
1-800-824-6396
Web site: www.lotuspress.com

154

Lotus Light carries a wide range of Ayurvedic supplies including herbs, soaps, oils, neti pots, and other equipment, as well as incense and teas.

Sushakti *(Wholesaler of Ayurvedic Rasayanas)*
1840 Iron Street, Suite C
Bellingham, WA 98225
1-888-SSHAKTI
Web site: www.ayurveda-sushakti.com

The Ayurvedic Institute
11311 Menaul NE
Albuquerque, NM 87112
(505) 291-9698
Fax: (505) 294-7572

The Ayurvedic Institute has traditional Ayurvedic and western herbs for sale. All herbs are organic, whenever possible, and are of the highest quality commercially available. Most herbs may be purchased in bulk quantities, subject to stock on hand. The institute is not a wholesaler, however. Some herbs from the Ayurvedic Institute are available in limited quantities only. Most are available in powdered form and some in whole form. There is a bulk discount of $1.50 per package on quantities of eight to fifteen ounces and a $4.00 discount per pound on quantities of one pound or more.

ESSENTIAL OILS

Liberty Naturals
8120 SE Stark Street
Portland, OR 97215
1-800-289-8427
Web site: www.libertynaturals.com

Best suppliers of pure essential oils at reasonable prices.

LEARNING RESOURCES

Sounds True
413 South Arthur Avenue
Louisville, CO 80027
1-888-303-9185
Fax: (303) 665-5292
E-mail: retail@soundstrue.com

Probably the best source of teaching tapes, videos, and CDs on spiritual and growth subjects. Among their best teaching tapes for those interested in Ayurvedic subjects are:

Meditation:
- *Awakening Compassion: Meditation Practice for Difficult Times* by Pema Chodren; six-cassette set.
- *Beginner's Mind: Three Classic Meditation Practices Especially for Beginners* taught by Jack Kornfield, Sharon Salzberg, and Shinzen Young; five-cassette set.
- *The Present Moment, a Retreat on Mindfulness* by Thich Nhat Hanh; six-cassette set.

Yoga:
- *Yoga Sanctuary* by Shiva Rea; the first complete hatha yoga class offered on CD; two-hour CD.
- *Yoga for Your Eyes: Natural Vision Improvement Exercises* by Meir Schneider; seventy-four minute video.
- *Mudra: Gestures of Power* by Sabrina Mesko; forty-five-minute video.

Mantras:
- *Mantras for Releasing Fear* by Shri Anandi Ma; ninety-minute cassette. This cassette offers four authentic chants for releasing fear and encouraging a peaceful spiritual state, using the ancient art of sacred sounds to influence body physiology and mental state.
- *The Power of Mantras: How to Use Sacred Words for Protection, Abundance, Creativity and Healing* by Thomas Ashley-Farrand; two-cassette set.
- *Mantra: Sacred Words of Power* by Thomas Ashley-Farrand; over eight hours of instruction; six-cassette set. Offers the most comprehensive course on Ayurvedic sound healing available anywhere.

Chakras:
- *The Chakra System* by Anodea Judith. How to learn chakra self-diagnosis and healing and how to balance your chakras. A complete self-teaching course on six cassettes.
- *Divine Singing* by Chaitanya Kabir. An innovative synthesis of music and spiritual practice in a nine-hour study course on six cassettes.
- Shambhala Publications. Contact at Horticultural Hall, 300 Massachusetts Avenue, Boston, MA 02115; 1-800-733-3000; Web site: www.shambhala.com. Probably the best source of wisdom publications in the United States. Send for their catalog.

156

AYURVEDA ON-LINE

Following is a guide to some of the best Web sites on all aspects of Ayurveda:

http://www.ayurveda.com
The Web site of Dr. Vasant Lad's institute, with many informative sections on Ayurveda, its history, their training courses, and herbal medicine supplies.

http://www.india-tourism.de/english/adressen/ayurveda.html
An Indian Web site with an excellent and comprehensible introduction
to Ayurveda, as well as a listing of the many places in India to visit,
including Ayurvedic health spas, retreats, and luxury hotels. A good
introduction to tourism in India, as well as to Ayurveda.

http://www.ayurveda-in.com/ayurveda.html
This is an excellent Web site that hosts all the Ayurvedic retreats and
treatment centers in Kerala, South India. Kerala is considered the great
center of Ayurveda in India today and it is also one of the most beautiful states in all India—lush, semitropical, covered with spice gardens,
edged by the fishing villages of the Indian Ocean, a total delight to visit.

http://www.farandawaydesign.com/inside.htm
An on-line magazine called *Inside Ayurveda: The Independent Journal of
Ayurvedic Health Care* that looks at current research, classical treatments,
and anything that involves the healing modes of Ayurveda. Good, interesting, and less reverent than many.

157

WEB SITES FOR
AYURVEDIC TREATMENT

http://www.health.indiamart.com/ayurveda/kapha-dosh.html
This is a general-information site on a number of alternative medicine
approaches, including Ayurveda. It is tied somewhat to the selling of
herbal medicines, but still a useful resource.

http://www.herbal-clinic.com/index.html
This is a site that is both charming and helpful, and it belongs to an
Ayurvedic physician's practice in Amadhabad, India. It lists many common medical conditions, treatments, and also allows you to E-mail the
doctor for advice.

http://www.aryaputra.com/home_contact/index.html
This is the Web site of an Ayurvedic M.D. in Akron, Ohio, who provides treatment according to the guidelines of Ayurveda, allied with
mainstream western treatment when patients request it.

http://www.pracsmart.com/AyurvedicHealthCare.html
This is an Australian Web site offering services such as a listing of practitioners, natural health information, and an Ayurvedic chat room. A
good way to contact others interested in Ayurveda.

AYURVEDIC EDUCATION

http://www.ayurveda.com
Dr. Vasant Lad's Ayurvedic Institute Web site with a complete listing of
the courses and Ayurvedic training available, plus extensive information
on Ayurveda, herbal medicine, treatments, and more. A very informative and helpful Web site.

http://www.ayurvedacollege.com/index.htm
The Web site of the California College of Ayurveda, the first nation-
ally recognized state-approved college for training in Ayurvedic medicine. This lists its courses, the work of its treatment center, and includes
a wide variety of Ayurvedic information.

http://www.vedicastrology.org
If you want to learn all about Vedic astrology, this is the site for you. It
includes educational opportunities, seminars, conferences, and whatever else is hot in the world of Vedic astrology. The American Council
of Vedic Astrology is based in New York.

http://www.himalayaninstitute.org/chh
The Himalayan Institute was founded by Swami Rama and offers
Ayurvedic and yoga teachings, courses, teacher training, and also an on-
line store of products and herbs.

http://www.floridavediccollege.edu/ayurveda/history.htm
The Vedic College of Florida offers many courses in Ayurvedic studies, from B.A. to Ph.D. This site gives full details of the courses available, tuition, registration, and E-mail for further information.

http://drhelenthomas.com/default.asp
This is the Web site of an Ayurvedic chiropractor who offers information and on-line workshops in Ayurvedic studies.

http://www.ayurvediccenter.com
The Web site of an Ayurvedic Treatment Center in Seattle.

AYURVEDIC HERBOLOGY

http://www.hindubooks.org/david_frawley/riverheaven/page22.htm
This is the Web site of David Frawley, an associate of Dr. Vasant Lad,
and it is packed with information about Ayurvedic herbs and their
healing abilities.

HERBAL SUPPLIERS

http://www.mountnebo.com/ayurvedic_herbs.htm
This is the Web site of a supplier of Ayurvedic herbs and medicines
based in Ohio. Their stock is extensive, their prices reasonable, and you
can order on-line if you choose.

http://www.banyanbotanicals.com/catreq.html
This is the Web site of associates of Dr. Vasant Lad, and it offers
Ayurvedic herbs, medicines, oils, essential oils, capsules, and pills. You
can order on-line or send for a catalog. A very complete stock list.

http://www.ayurveda.com/herbstore.htm
This is the on-line herb store of the Ayurvedic Institute, where you can
browse through the extensive stock of finest quality herbs and make
your purchases on-line. Its stock also includes other Ayurvedic products such as *malas* or prayer beads, neti pots, soaps, oils, and more.

http://www.greenking.com/ayurved.html
This is the Ayurvedic section of Green King's herbal products in which
all the standard Ayurvedic herbal medicinals are available in a tincture
form.

http://www.mapi.com
A listing of all the supplies, herbs, medicinal oils, and complete
Ayurvedic paraphernalia from one of the primary resources in the
United States.

http://www.indistores.com/indiherbs/index1.htm
Another excellent source of Ayurvedic herbs, plus on-line consultation
with Ayurvedic physicians.

YOGA

http://yogadirectory.com
This is the site for everything you ever wanted to know about finding yoga lessons and teachers, schools of yoga, education in yoga, and so on. The biggest and best.

http://www.viniyoga.com
This is the site of the American Viniyoga Institute, which offers teaching and teacher training in Viniyoga with classes at various locations in the United States.

http://comnet.org/iynaus
This is the Web site of the Iyengar Yoga Institute, probably the most famous of all the great teachers of yoga. You can find schools and teachers from this site.

160

BOOKS

http://www.amazon.com
The first, biggest, and best of the on-line bookstores, which also has audiotapes and videotapes, music, and other kinds of shopping.

http://www.yogabooks.net
The book-supplying branch of Lotus Light with a list of all the main yoga books available from this publisher.

AYURVEDA FOR
SPECIFIC CONDITIONS

http://www.veda-vyasa.com
This is a Web site made by an Ayurvedic practitioner in India who treats diabetes successfully with Ayurvedic herbs.

http://health.indiamart.com/ayurveda/common-problems/
constipation.html
This is the traditional Ayurvedic approach to treating constipation.

http://health.indiamart.com/ayurveda/common-
problems/arthritis-jointpain.html
This is the traditional Ayurvedic approach to treating arthritis.

http://health.indiamart.com/ayurveda/common-problems/
common-cold.html
This is the traditional Ayurvedic approach to the common cold.

AUTHOR CONTACT INFORMATION

Frena Gray-Davidson can be contacted at fregrayda@hotmail.com or   161
visit her Web site at www.geocities.com/hotsprings/1159.

BIBLIOGRAPHY

GENERAL

Chopra, Deepak, M.D. *Perfect Health*. New York: Harmony Books, 1991.

Frawley, David. *Ayurvedic Healing*. Salt Lake City, Utah: Morson Publishing, 1989.

————. *Ayurveda and the Mind*. Twin Lakes, Wis.: Lotus Press, 1997.

Frawley, David, and Vasant Lad. *The Yoga of Herbs: An Ayurvedic Guide to Herbal Medicine*. Santa Fe, N.M.: Lotus Press, 1988.

Gerson, Scott. *Ayurveda: The Ancient Indian Healing Art*. Rockport, Mass.: Element Books, 1993.

Heyn, B. *Ayurveda: India's Art of Natural Medicine and Life Extension*. Rochester, Vt.: Healing Arts Press, 1988.

Lad, Vasant. *Ayurveda, the Science of Self-Healing*. Santa Fe, N.M.: Lotus Press, 1984.

Svoboda, Robert. *Prakruti: Your Ayurvedic Constitution*. Albuquerque, N.M.: Geocom Press, 1988.

Tiwari, M. *A Life of Balance: The Complete Guide to Ayurvedic Nutrition*. Rochester, Vt.: Healing Arts Press, 1995.

YOGA

Feurstein, Georg. *The Shambhala Encyclopedia of Yoga.* Boston, Mass.: Shambhala Publications, 2000.

———. *The Shambhala Guide to Yoga.* Boston, Mass.: Shambhala Publications, 1996.

Iyengar, B. K. S. *The Tree of Yoga.* Boston, Mass.: Shambhala Publications, 1989.

MEDITATION

Chodren, P. *The Wisdom of No Escape.* Boston, Mass.: Shambhala Publications, 1991.

———. *Start Where You Are.* Boston, Mass.: Shambhala Publications, 1994.

———. *When Things Fall Apart.* Boston, Mass.: Shambhala Publications, 1996.

———. *Awakening Loving-Kindness.* Boston, Mass.: Shambhala Publications, 1996.

Goldstein, J. *Seeking the Heart of Wisdom: The Path of Insight Meditation.* Boston, Mass.: Shambhala Publications, 2001.

Johnson, W. *The Posture of Meditation.* Boston, Mass.: Shambhala Publications, 1996. (Note: This small but valuable book is a practical guide for meditators of all traditions.)

Nairn, R. *What Is Meditation?* Boston, Mass.: Shambhala Publications, 2000.

Salzberg, S. *Lovingkindness: The Revolutionary Art of Happiness.* Boston, Mass.: Shambhala Publications, 1997.

ESSENTIAL OILS

Lavabre, M. *Aromatherapy Workbook.* Rochester, Vt.: Healing Arts Press, 1990.

Lawless, J. *The Illustrated Encyclopedia of Essential Oils.* Rockport, Mass.: Element Books, 1995.

Ody, P. *The Complete Medicinal Herbal.* New York: D&K, 1993.

Tisserand, M. *Aromatherapy for Women.* U.K.: Thorsons, 1985.

Tisserand, R. *The Art of Aromatherapy.* U.K.: C. W. Daniel, 1985.

Valnet, J. *The Practice of Aromatherapy.* U.K.: C. W. Daniel, 1982.

Worwood, V. A. *The Complete Guide to Aromatherapy and Essential Oils.* Palo Alto, Calif.: New World, 1996.

INDEX

169

M

175

Q

R

S

W

Y